'I wish this book had existed when I was younger, in the midst of pain and uncertainty, searching for answers. It might have been the guide I needed while navigating the long road to diagnosis and understanding my own body. May this book provide some guidance and support on your endo journey.'

—Ellie Angel Mobbs

'A useful, usable companion for all those with endometriosis or caring for someone with endometriosis.'

—Professor Jason Abbott, Professor of Obstetrics and Gynaecology, UNSW Sydney Australia

'A much-needed evidence-based, accessible book for those living with endometriosis and challenged by fertility.'

—Professor Luk Rombauts, Past President of the World Endometriosis Society

'The impact of endometriosis on the lives and wellbeing of women is profound. Despite this, many aspects of the disease are poorly understood, and high quality treatments are lacking. Maree Davenport shines a light on this complex disease with informed input from a wide range of stakeholders. Essential reading for anyone wanting to understand more about living with endometriosis.'

—Professor Peter AW Rogers, Professor of Women's Health Research, University of Melbourne; Director of Research, Royal Women's Hospital; Founding Director and current Board Member, Jean Hailes Foundation.

'The only way we can affect improved Endometriosis care is by brave people sharing their stories. Congratulations to Maree Davenport and her contributors for explaining the challenges, providing context, understanding and advocating for change in this book that will positively impact many people's lives.'

—Professor Louise Hull

'This book will be life changing for women of all ages. It will help end the silent suffering that's been the "women's lot" for generations.'

—A/Prof Magdalena Simonis AM

The Australian Guide to Living Well with Endometriosis

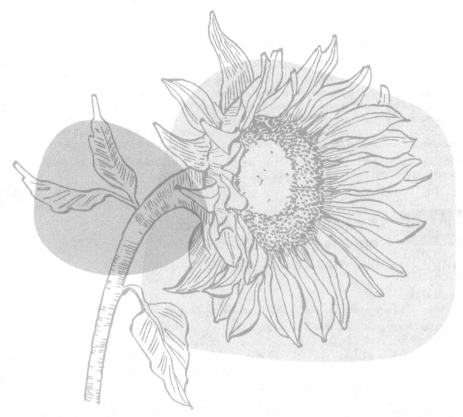

The Australian Guide to Living Well with Endometriosis

Maree Davenport

WILEY

First published 2025 by John Wiley & Sons Australia, Ltd

© John Wiley & Sons Australia, Ltd 2025

All rights reserved, including rights for text and data mining and training of artificial intelligence technologies or similar technologies. Except as permitted under the *Australian Copyright Act 1968* (for example, a fair dealing for the purposes of study, research, criticism or review) no part of this publication may be reproduced, stored in a retrieval system, or transmitted, in any form or by any means, electronic, mechanical, photocopying, recording or otherwise. Advice on how to obtain permission to reuse material from this title is available at http://www.wiley.com/go/permissions.

The right of Maree Davenport to be identified as the author of *The Australian Guide to Living Well with Endometriosis* has been asserted in accordance with law.

ISBN: 978-1-394-29590-6

A catalogue record for this book is available from the National Library of Australia

Registered Office
John Wiley & Sons Australia, Ltd. Level 4, 600 Bourke Street, Melbourne, VIC 3000, Australia

For details of our global editorial offices, customer services, and more information about Wiley products visit us at www.wiley.com.

Wiley also publishes its books in a variety of electronic formats and by print-on-demand. Some content that appears in standard print versions of this book may not be available in other formats.

Trademarks: Wiley and the Wiley logo are trademarks or registered trademarks of John Wiley & Sons, Inc. and/or its affiliates in the United States and other countries and may not be used without written permission. All other trademarks are the property of their respective owners. John Wiley & Sons, Inc. is not associated with any product or vendor mentioned in this book.

Limit of Liability/Disclaimer of Warranty
While the publisher and author have used their best efforts in preparing this work, they make no representations or warranties with respect to the accuracy or completeness of the contents of this work and specifically disclaim all warranties, including without limitation any implied warranties of merchantability or fitness for a particular purpose. No warranty may be created or extended by sales representatives, written sales materials or promotional statements for this work. This work is sold with the understanding that the publisher is not engaged in rendering professional services. The advice and strategies contained herein may not be suitable for your situation. You should consult with a specialist where appropriate. The fact that an organisation, website, or product is referred to in this work as a citation and/or potential source of further information does not mean that the publisher and author endorse the information or services the organisation, website, or product may provide or recommendations it may make. Further, readers should be aware that websites listed in this work may have changed or disappeared between when this work was written and when it is read. Neither the publisher nor author shall be liable for any loss of profit or any other commercial damages, including but not limited to special, incidental, consequential, or other damages.

We do not accept any liability for any injury, loss or damage caused by use of the information provided in our book or on the website. The information may include the views or recommendations of third parties and does not necessarily reflect the views of the authors and website owners, who are not medically trained, nor do they claim to be.

This book contains links to websites to help you find more information. While the author is careful in selecting the websites, we are not responsible for and do not necessarily endorse their information. You need to make your own decisions about the accuracy, currency and reliability of information in linked websites.

Cover design by Wiley
Cover and part opener image: © samiradragonfly/Adobe Stock

Set in 11.5/13.5pt ITC BerkeleyStd, Straive, Chennai, India.

SKYE34AE5A7-E8C1-4F83-BF77-1F609168A9A8_022025

Disclaimer

While I've made every effort to ensure that the information in this book is accurate and informative, it does not take the place of professional or medical advice.

Do not use this information:
- to diagnose, treat, cure or prevent any disease
- for therapeutic purposes
- as a substitute for the advice of a health professional.

To my daughter Brianna, niece Alicia and all the incredible endo warriors, I am deeply grateful for your unwavering resilience, strength, persistence, patience, and courage in the face of daily challenges.

This book is a labour of love, intended to serve as a guiding light through the lenses familiar to me — the healthcare system, gender equality, politics, policy, advocacy and empowerment.

My sincere hope is that this book will help you live well with endometriosis and cultivate a community of compassion that recognises your individual needs.

I also aim to educate those providing care; encourage respectful collaboration with their patients; and better address this life-altering, chronic and currently incurable condition.

This continues the legacy of the late Professor David Healy, and I dedicate this book to him, almost 30 years after he first lobbied me about a life-defining, gendered disease called endometriosis.

Contents

Foreword   xvii

About the author   xix

Introduction   xxi

PART I | Tune in: Understanding endo   1

1   What is endometriosis?   3
Are heavy, painful periods normal?   4
Symptoms to look out for   5
Genetics and gastrointestinal issues   7
What about adenomyosis?   8
Does endometriosis have different stages or levels?   8
Endo myths and facts   11
What causes endometriosis?   13
What might be going on in the body?   13

2   Understanding the pain and fatigue   17
Understanding pelvic pain   17
Unwelcome friends   25
Am I more likely to have other chronic conditions as well
  as endo?   25

PART II | Track, Tell, Test: Getting a diagnosis   27

3   How do I find a name for my pain?   29
Endo is more common than you think   29
The journey to get tested and diagnosed   30

Track your symptom impact 31
Heavy menstrual bleeding 35

4 What kind of doctor do you need? 39
What symptoms do GPs look for in endometriosis? 40
Creating your care team and plan 41
Professor Danielle Mazza AM on how a GP diagnoses endo 44
A referral to the gynaecologist 47
Dr Tarana Lucky on what to expect at the gyno 48

5 What to expect from examinations and tests 51
Rachel Andrew on preparing for a physical exam 52
Pelvic examination 53
Medical imaging 54
Ultrasound 54
Imagendo 55
Associate Professor Magdalena Simonis AM on symptoms and testing 58
Dr Tarana Lucky on tests at the gyno 60

PART III | Treat: Considering your options 63

6 What are my treatment options? 65
Over-the-counter medications 65
Analgesics 66
Non-steroidal anti-inflammatories 66
Palmitoylethanolamide (PEA) 66
Prescription medications 66
Why are they prescribing the pill? 68
Hormone treatment options 69
Traditional and alternative options 76

7 Considering surgery 81
Laparoscopic surgery 81
Hysterectomy 85

8 Fertility and infertility 89
How does endo impact fertility? 90
What to expect from a fertility specialist 92
Fertility treatment options 93

Starting the IVF process   94
Professor Luk Rombauts on how endo impacts fertility   95
Dr Samantha Mooney on treatment options   97
Dealing with the tough stuff   102

9   Multidisciplinary care   107
Biopsychosocial approaches   107
Stephanie O'Kane on supporting patients' varied needs   110
Allied health   114
Akaiti James on her approach to holistic care   116
Rachel Andrew with the lowdown on physio below
   the belt   118
Acupuncture for endo   122
Osteopathy for endometriosis   123
Dr Lisa Gadd on different endo therapies   124
Benefits of massage for endometriosis   125
Psychological support   127
Physical activity and exercise   127
Mind-body practices   128
Pacing activities   128
Stress management   128
Sleep hygiene   128
Emotional support   128
Integrative health   131
Body image   132

10   Relationships   139
Dads as endo supporters   141
Endometriosis and its impact on intimate relationships   142
Educational resources   145
Couples counselling   145
Endometriosis and its impact on family planning   146
Sex and intimacy   147
Intimacy beyond sexuality   147
Daily life and responsibilities   147
Social isolation   148
Support networks   148

PART IV | Try it out: Holistic lifestyle and self-care 149

11 Lifestyle and self-care 151
'Nothing about us without us' 152

12 Diet and nutrition 155
Are you what you eat? 155
The daily dozen 157
Adapting your diet to what works for you 158
Low-FODMAP diet 159
Anti-inflammatory diet 161
Omega-3 fatty acids 162
To soy or not to soy? 162
Gut microbiota and endometriosis 163
Antioxidants and gut health 164
Benefits of fermented foods 165
Dr Eliza Colgrave on balancing diet and exercise 165
Heal. Nourish. Support. Balance. 169

13 Exercise for endo 173
Rolling with life's curveballs: Lisa's story 174
Dr Lisa Gadd's endometriosis stretches to attain 'living
health' 176
Protecting with abdominal exercises 179

14 Rest and recuperation 187
Listening to what your body needs: Ellie's story 187
Fatigue and Spoon Theory 188
Cold therapy 192
Heat therapy 196

PART V | Take it on: Know your rights 199

15 School and work 201
Endo girls 202
Teachers need to step up 204
LongSTEPPP 205
School education 206
Endo gendernomics 207
About Bloody Time 211
Endometriosis and the workplace 214

16 Medical misogyny 231

How the medical world excludes and ignores women+ 232
End Gender Bias survey 233
GP gender pay gap 237
Bias in research funding 237

17 Intersectionality and inclusion in care 239

Aboriginal and Torres Strait Islanders 240
Dr Maryam Moradi on increasing awareness
of endometriosis 249
LGBTQIA+ 250

PART VI | Take action: Global efforts 257

18 What's the future of endo research and policy? 259

National Endometriosis Clinical Scientific Trials Registry 259
Professor Jason Abbott on the need for multi-disciplinary
support for people with endometriosis 260
Parliamentary Friends of Endometriosis Awareness 262
National Action Plan on Endometriosis 263
Endometriosis and pelvic pain clinics 263
Global endo efforts 267
The gift of philanthropy 270

Acknowledgements 273

Resources 279

References 295

Index 317

Foreword

The Governor-General of the Commonwealth of Australia Her Excellency the Honourable Ms Sam Mostyn AC.

For many years, it has been my privilege to work for equality for women. During that time, I have learned from so many women of the devastating pain and misunderstanding that accompanies endometriosis.

On the good news front, this dreadful, debilitating disease is now, more than ever before, the subject of open conversations, improved understanding and better-funded research. In the last decade, more and more women have spoken up and spoken out about their experiences with this insidious disease. More and more women are breaking the silence and lighting the way for those who live with endometriosis.

And there are many of them. One million or more Australian women and girls live with endometriosis, many of them still burdened by the myths, silences and misrepresentations that have surrounded this disease for generations. I know so many of these women, young and old. The Australian Institute of Health and Welfare tells us that the number of women diagnosed by the age of 50 has risen to one in seven.

For many, a comprehensive diagnosis is often the answer to a question that has dogged their health and wellbeing for years.

Especially when, on average, diagnosis takes 6.5 years—longer for women in regional and rural areas and in disadvantaged communities. Receiving a diagnosis after years of pain and suffering can be the beginning of a better life.

This book is part of that journey. It offers support and affirmation as well as practical insights and empirical, evidence-based conclusions. It breaks new ground in sharing the game-changing advances in endometriosis health, infertility and research. To the women who share their own experiences here with great courage and honesty, my heart goes out in gratitude. You represent so many of the women in my life who share your journey.

This book is an expression not only of medical rigour and bold advocacy but, fundamentally, of care. Care for the many who are suffering. Care for the networks of frontline workers and health professionals who themselves are giving constantly with outstretched hands and thoughtful counsel.

My hope is that in the years ahead, endometriosis will be less of a menace to health and happiness. Instead, it may become a cause to celebrate medical breakthroughs, our respect for women and the widening circles of care that encompass every woman and girl.

About the author

Maree Davenport has advocated for women+'s health for over 30 years. She was the youngest woman elected to the Parliament of Victoria at age 28 and the first to have a baby while serving. She was appointed as chair of the government's Health Policy Committee and Parliamentary Secretary for Health. Maree holds a Master of Leadership specialising in gender equality, diversity and inclusion. She also has tertiary qualifications in property, communications, risk (GIA) and governance (AICD), and is an accredited mediator (NMAS), specialising in workplace disputes and Gender Equality Action Plans.

She is passionate about endometriosis and a strong advocate. She is committed to reducing diagnostic delay; improving ultrasound and magnetic resonance imaging (MRI) access to avoid invasive surgery; preserving fertility; and empowering person-centred, multidisciplinary health and self-care.

She has shared the life-defining challenges of endometriosis and adenomyosis through her daughter, Brianna, who developed symptoms at the age of eight. The challenges affect all facets of her life.

Brianna is committed to helping other endo warriors and as a nurse, working through COVID-19 in Monash Health's emergency department. She understands the challenges with fertility and pregnancy risk and is now a fertility nurse. She and her husband, Daniel, a paramedic, welcomed their son Oliver in August 2022.

Maree's niece Alicia was diagnosed with endometriosis after investigation of fertility issues, in 2023 and, after undergoing treatment, welcomed daughter Margot with her husband Nick in May 2024.

Maree Davenport was chief executive officer of an endometriosis charity for a year from March 2023. During that time, she elevated media coverage and government action, resulting in successful awareness campaigns leading to federal government funding and subsidies through Medicare. She previously served as chair on the Board and on the Federal Department of Health's Endometriosis Expert Advisory Group.

She is on the organising committee for the World Congress on Endometriosis (Sydney 2025), chair of the Patient Liaison Committee, and an organiser of the inaugural Endo Warrior community day.

She has three children and is 'Nanree' to three grandchildren. She lives in Melbourne with husband Marcus, and Zac and Rocky, their fur babies.

Introduction

Endo-mee-tree-osis...the sound of it is something quite atrocious.

Endometriosis is hard to say and awful to live with.

Thank you for taking the time to read this book about living with a chronic, whole-of-body inflammatory disease, which is incurable; life-defining; adversely impacts fertility, body image and sex lives; and, in general, involves pain that stops you from fully participating in the life you choose to lead.

Know this from the outset: women+ living with endometriosis are strong, resilient, organised and have an endurance well beyond the realms of normal capacity.

Imagine if men had life-impacting pain for weeks at a time, found sex painful, pee and poo problematic, and constantly felt sick and tired. Governments, researchers and philanthropists would have invested in finding a cure for these symptoms decades ago.

If men walked in the impractical, uncomfortable shoes of the one in seven women+ diagnosed with endometriosis (endo) by their fiftieth birthday, and faced poor body image arising from bloating, they would understand why so many of these women+ are anxious and depressed.

In Australia, endo is as common as diabetes, affecting 14 per cent of girls and women+. The World Health Organization estimates the condition affects around 190 million reproductive-age girls and women+ globally. It states: 'Addressing endometriosis will empower those affected by it by supporting their human right to the highest standard of sexual and reproductive health, quality of life and overall well-being.'

Women+ are at a disadvantage in a medical system designed by men, specifically for the Reference Man in 1974, a theoretical person who has 'normal' characteristics. Meaning *he* is between 20 and 30 years of age, weighs 70 kilos, is 170 cm tall, and is Western European or North American.

Until recently, healthcare data and drug trials have used this man to decide what works for women+'s health and diseases, as well as safe medication doses. Female medication has been developed and tested on male subjects.

Endometriosis is an enigma

We do not understand the cause of endometriosis, and we lack effective therapies to treat it. It is not solely a complex gynaecological or reproductive health condition, and it is frustrating to see it reduced to period pain and heat packs.

Despite being first described over a century ago, many aspects of endometriosis, including its development, progression, the pain it causes and its impact on fertility, remain poorly understood. The so-called 'gold standard' definitive diagnosis remains dependent on invasive laparoscopic surgery, even with advances in ultrasound and magnetic resonance imaging (MRI) technology.

In Australia, too many general practitioners (GPs), gynaecologists and nurses in schools, hospitals and health centres are unaware of endometriosis symptoms. This delays diagnosis and significantly impacts physical and mental health, quality of life, capacity to study and work, social life and intimate relationships.

Endometriosis is the third-leading cause of non-fatal disease burden among females, and each year it results in 40 500 endometriosis-related hospitalisations. It can occur in girls as young as eight. Pregnancy is not a 'cure', it simply reduces and disrupts the estrogen that feeds the lesions, while the woman+ is pregnant and breastfeeding. For many, symptoms persist beyond menopause and hysterectomy. This is a lifelong, life-defining, gendered disease.

Hippocrates, who was known as the 'father of medicine', described women+'s health and pelvic health issues as a 'wandering womb', believing the uterus dislodged and moved around the body. In a way, modern science confirmed his theory. Endometriosis is a system-wide hormonal disease in which cells like those found in the uterus or womb grow in the wrong places. This results in inflammation and a cycle of healing and scarring.

It is challenging to diagnose, treat and manage symptoms that vary from day to day, month to month and 'flare-up' without warning. To borrow from John Lennon, 'Life is what happens to you while you're busy making other plans'. Endo symptoms do not consider your life's plans.

Worrying about flare-ups can derail special events, social engagements, sports, work and study commitments. The stress from this worry impacts the nervous system, and growing evidence indicates this leads to pain and sensitivity. Chronic pain develops over time because of central sensitisation or pain hypersensitivity.

Pain is exhausting—it affects sleep, and the medications aimed at easing it can make you feel sick, drowsy and, worse, can cause addiction. All of this fatigue causes psychological distress.

The average time to diagnose endometriosis is six and a half years, and it can be even longer depending on where you live. It is not fair that people in rural and regional areas are disadvantaged by 'postcode lottery'. New ways to screen for endometriosis and more effective therapies to treat it are urgently needed. Early recognition of symptoms and timely intervention are crucial.

As you will read, it is a heartbreaking yet consistent theme among those who have shared their personal journey with endometriosis that, when they sought medical help, even while exhibiting severe pain, heavy menstrual bleeding, and bowel and urination issues, they were dismissed, belittled, ignored and their symptoms and suffering minimised.

Endometriosis is a political issue

In 2017, the Australian Government apologised to those living with endometriosis at the launch of the nonpartisan Parliamentary Friends of Endometriosis Awareness. The Minister for Health and Aged Care, the Hon. Greg Hunt, said:

> *On behalf of all of those in parliament and all of those who have been responsible for our medical system, I apologise. This condition should have been acknowledged at an earlier time in a more powerful way and will never be forgotten again.*

This led to the development and funding of the Australian National Action Plan on Endometriosis (NAPE). The five-year plan expired in 2023 and the federal government has not committed to a new plan or confirmed ongoing funding beyond the programs already in progress.

Substantial new and ongoing funding is urgently needed for research investment. We need long-term, renewed and targeted efforts to understand the impact of endometriosis on girls and women+, their health, fertility and economic disadvantage.

In particular, priority populations face intersectional disadvantage, including Aboriginal and Torres Strait Islanders, those from culturally and linguistically diverse and religiously conservative traditions. Menstruation and reproductive women+'s health are often taboo and, therefore, not discussed, or even actively avoided. Young girls and those in rural and regional areas need access to education, and the LGBTQIA+ community urgently needs barriers to healthcare access removed.

We need to teach girls and women+ to advocate for themselves

Girls and women+ should be encouraged and supported to advocate for themselves as the person at the centre of their multidisciplinary and integrated care. They deserve confidence in self-management of symptoms, and should be forearmed with tools to do so at home, school or work.

The personal endo journeys we share, the cold, hard reality of living with a warm heat pack; endo bloat; heavy bleeding at any time of the month; digestive issues; the impact on intimate relationships; the roller-coaster of fertility; heartbreak of pregnancy loss; reduced social, work and financial security; the 'endo gender pay gap'; and disrupted social and community life are a call to action.

We need to inform, advise and educate the community as a whole and form a safety net around girls and women+ experiencing pelvic pain and symptoms that might be endometriosis, its 'ugly sister' adenomyosis, polycystic ovary syndrome (PCOS) or be related to their bowel or bladder.

When I say 'we', I mean me as the author in partnership with the contributors to this book; the 'endo warriors' from all ages and stages of life who share their experiences, as well as the doctors and professors, researchers and other health providers who share their expertise.

We aim to empower you with up-to-date, trustworthy, evidence-based, medically sound and useful information so that you can be heard, understood, supported and, importantly, validated. We want to grow your confidence in developing action plans and knowing when you need to escalate medical intervention.

You'll learn about the four D's of endometriosis, and here are the first couple. Research from the Universities of Adelaide and Monash of women+ living with endometriosis found 65.8 per cent reported period pain (dysmenorrhoea) and 61.1 per cent reported painful sex (dyspareunia) despite medical and surgical intervention. In the previous three months, 82.7 per cent reported chronic pelvic pain. On average, they had sought help from three different health practitioner specialties in the previous 12 months for their endometriosis. Unfortunately, medical misogyny, gaslighting and the postcode lottery result in disparities in health practitioners taking symptoms seriously enough to refer to specialists.

The endo journey

We will guide you through the complicated spiderweb of referral pathways to help manage pain, fertility challenges and life-impacting consequences. We will show you how to foster an integrative health approach involving gynaecologists, pain specialists, dietitians and allied and complementary health professionals, mental health support and other healthcare providers.

You will also learn about informed decision making, a fundamental aspect of patient-centred healthcare that involves open communication between patients and healthcare practitioners to make decisions dependent on each unique circumstance, taking into consideration beliefs and familial, social and personal priorities. This is particularly important for those from culturally, linguistically and religiously diverse communities.

We aim to equip healthcare professionals and practitioners with the skills and knowledge to diagnose, treat and help manage the confronting symptoms of their patients.

Nothing tells a story better than one written using the words of those who have lived the experience, and we are grateful to the many brave and diverse voices who have shared their vulnerabilities, emotions and impacts of persistent pelvic pain and other experiences.

They share strategies to empower you to live well in every aspect of your life and embrace it fully and richly so you can travel along the 'yellow brick road' and not get lost in the weeds. We aim to do this with humour and respect for those with chronic health issues. We will explore research into intricate interactions between genetics, lifestyle and environment, and how treatments can improve health outcomes.

Even if you have not personally experienced endometriosis symptoms, we aim to educate through cold plunge immersion, taking you from your ambient, pleasant comfort zone into the world of medical misogyny and the 'P party' filled with pain, periods, poo, pee and painful sex.

If you care for someone impacted by this relentless condition, we aim to empower you as parents, partners, family, workmates, community members and sports teams to advocate for them.

Endo activism

The term 'endo warrior' appears throughout the book; this has become the catchcry of the movement within the endometriosis community to combat stigma and promote awareness. It emphasises the strength and courage of those living with endometriosis, portraying them as warriors fighting against a condition that is often misunderstood or dismissed.

Yellow has been associated with endometriosis awareness campaigns since 1980. In March 1993, Endometriosis Awareness Week began in Milwaukee, Wisconsin, and today, international Endometriosis Awareness Month is in March each year.

I am honoured to be on the organising committee for the 2025 World Congress on Endometriosis in Sydney, Australia. Researchers from across the globe will share their work aimed at improving diagnosis and treatment, and finding a cure. The World Endometriosis Society also focuses on the impacts it has on those living with endometriosis, including medical, surgical and fertility; allied, complementary and alternative treatment; pain mechanisms and management; and people, policy and politics in endometriosis.

I welcome you on this journey of awareness, and sincerely hope this book contributes to bringing the discussion of endometriosis and the associated symptoms into the public discourse so women+ experiencing this debilitating disease can get the diagnosis, treatment and understanding they deserve.

I have chosen the sunflower to represent yellow, the colour for 'endo warriors', and because the flowers follow the sun as they grow. When they reach maturity, their stems become fixed, stuck. This symbolises the life-defining impact of endometriosis for women+. Without a timely diagnosis, treatment and fertility advice, too many become impacted by the life-long disease, which invades every facet of their lives, like the endo lesions.

Let's begin.

PART I

Tune in

Understanding endo

CHAPTER 1

What is endometriosis?

Endometriosis is the presence of normal tissue in abnormal places.

The monthly menstrual cycle occurs when the hormone estrogen signals the tissue in the innermost layer of the uterus, the endometrium, to plump up with blood and thicken so that it can support the implantation of a fertilised egg. When a pregnancy doesn't occur, the lining breaks down and leaves the body; this is a period.

In endometriosis, similar cells to this lining grow outside of the uterus, and respond to the hormone signals from estrogen just like the lining of the uterus does—they grow and bleed with the menstrual cycle. Endometriosis commonly involves the pelvic area (below the belt) and impacts the ovaries and fallopian tubes. It can affect nearby organs, including the bowel, rectum and bladder, and it can also affect other organs outside the pelvic cavity.

This causes chronic, long-term inflammation, which is your body's defence system's response to the presence of those endometriosis cells. Unlike normal endometrium, this tissue doesn't leave the body during menstruation, leading to inflammation and scar tissue formation. These are called lesions and adhesions. Both cause pain in endometriosis but are different.

Lesions are patches of endometrial-like tissue that vary in size and colour (clear, brown, black, blue, red or white). They can be small, flat, raised or nodular, and are usually found in the pelvic area, but can occasionally appear in organs like the brain or lungs. There are three main types of lesions:

1. superficial peritoneal lesions: small patches on the peritoneum (the lining of the abdominal cavity)
2. endometriomas (chocolate cysts): cysts on the ovaries filled with thick brown fluid
3. deep infiltrating endometriosis (DIE): aggressive lesions affecting deeper tissues.

Adhesions are thick bands of scar tissue that bind organs together. They result from inflammation and injuries, not from hormonal responses like lesions. Adhesions can be caused by endometriosis, surgery, infection or other tissue damage.

The presence of endometriosis in the pelvis can cause several different symptoms, including pain and trouble achieving pregnancy.

Are heavy, painful periods normal?

It is important to be able to distinguish between normal menstrual cramps and endometriosis pain. The following five factors might help you start to identify whether your periods are within the normal range or if there is something more going on.

1. Timing and duration

Normal menstrual cramps typically begin one to two days before a period starts and subside a few days after bleeding begins.

Endometriosis pain often starts as many as one to two weeks before a period and can last throughout and even after the period ends. The pain is more constant than cramping.

2. Severity

Menstrual cramps are usually mild to moderate in severity and can be managed with over-the-counter pain medication.

Endometriosis pain is often described as severe, debilitating and not relieved by typical pain medication. It can disrupt daily activities.

3. Cyclical vs non-cyclical

Menstrual cramps follow a cyclical pattern, occurring only around the time blood and other matter are discharged from the uterus during menstruation. The menstrual cycle begins on the first day of your period and ends when your next period begins.

Endometriosis pain can be constant, with heightened pain during menstrual periods but also between cycles.

4. Progression

Period cramps tend to be relatively consistent from cycle to cycle.

Endometriosis pain often progressively worsens over time as the condition advances if it is left untreated.

5. Other symptoms

Normal periods may involve bloating, breast tenderness and mild back pain.

Endometriosis has additional symptoms such as painful intercourse, heavy bleeding, gastrointestinal issues (diarrhoea, constipation, nausea) and infertility.

Symptoms to look out for

While not an inclusive list, the following highlights the varied symptoms people with endometriosis may experience.

Pain is the most reported symptom of endometriosis. The location of the pain will depend on the inflammation and scar tissue, as well as the time of the menstrual cycle. Some people will have multiple symptoms.

Pelvic pain

Women+ with endometriosis often feel pain 'below the belt' during menstruation and ovulation. Some women+ experience this for a long time (chronic pelvic pain). The following symptoms can be some of the most obvious and common signs of endometriosis.

Painful periods and cramps

This is called dysmenorrhea. Severe pain before and during periods from an early age, even as young as eight, can be one of the first indicators of endometriosis. These cramp-like pains may extend into the abdomen or lower back.

Heavy menstrual bleeding or irregular periods

The technical definition for heavy menstrual bleeding is anything exceeding 80 millilitres. This is hard to measure, so be guided by how often you change your sanitary products—if it is hourly or close to it, visit your GP. Other symptoms include getting up during the night to change period products, passing clots (especially if they're bigger than a 50-cent coin) or feeling dizzy or tired. Women+ with endometriosis may experience heavy menstrual bleeding or irregular menstrual periods lasting more than seven days.

Heavy menstrual bleeding affects a quarter of girls and women+ from when they start periods until menopause (the 'reproductive years'). Over two-thirds of them are iron deficient.

Bleeding between menstrual periods

Spotting or bleeding between menstrual periods can be a symptom of endometriosis.

Pain when toileting

This is called dyschezia for poo and dysuria for wee. Lesions and adhesions can grow around the bladder, bowel and rectum. Inflammation can cause issues with frequent weeing, constipation, diarrhoea and the feeling that poo is 'stuck'. This may be worse around your period; for many, it happens frequently and all month.

Pain during or after sex

This is called dyspareunia. The pain is most commonly described as occurring during intercourse rather than at the start or end, and is often more severe with deep penetration. In one study, pain during or after sex was reported by 92 per cent of their sample of women+ with endometriosis.

Pain in other areas

Endometriosis has also been found outside the pelvis, which can result in gastrointestinal issues, fatigue and pain in other areas of the body, such as joints.

Leg pain

Endometriosis lesions can affect the nerves that lead to the legs, causing pain, numbness or tingling down the legs. This could affect any of the following areas:
- joints: back, knees, hips, hands and feet can be sore, stiff and achy, and they can be burning or numb; there is also an increased risk of rheumatoid arthritis

6 The Australian Guide to Living Well with Endometriosis

- shoulders: lesions can grow on the diaphragm (in rare cases), causing referred pain in the shoulder area during menstruation
- chest: lesions have been found growing on the lungs (in very rare cases), causing chest pain or a chronic cough
- headaches/migraines: there is a higher risk of migraines and headaches, possibly due to the inflammatory nature of the condition.

Digestive and gastrointestinal symptoms

Gastrointestinal symptoms can also be common with of endometriosis, and this presents with a range of symptoms to watch out for.

Endo belly

Distended, swollen bloating can occur any time of the month, but is most common around ovulation and your period. Sometimes this is accompanied by nausea, vomiting, toileting problems, cramps or stomach pain, indigestion, heartburn, gas pains and farting, constipation or diarrhoea. It is always unwelcome and has a negative impact on body image.

Many women+ with endo initially seek help from gastroenterologists and are diagnosed with irritable bowel syndrome (IBS), delaying the diagnosis of endometriosis. It is really hard to find the reason for bloating when the small intestine is about 6 metres long; the large (wider, not longer) intestine runs for 1.5 metres, and it includes the rectum, which is around 12 centimetres. Sometimes, endometriosis lesions can be near the bowel, or on it, but inflammation causes discomfort regardless of the cause.

A recent study on biopsychosocial health outcomes for adult women+ with co-occurring endometriosis and IBS symptoms found individuals were 'inclined to exhibit more complex change trajectories in psychological distress, magnification, and fatigue over time, with a trend towards worse outcomes overall' than those with endometriosis alone.

Genetics and gastrointestinal issues

A 2023 study from the University of Queensland's Institute for Molecular Bioscience by Yang et al. involving highly respected researchers Professor Grant Montgomery and Professor Gita Mishra found genetic risk factors are shared among several gastrointestinal disorders, including IBS, peptic ulcer disease, gastro-oesophageal reflux disease, inflammatory bowel disease and endometriosis.

Women+ with endometriosis were found to be twice as likely to have an IBS diagnosis compared to women+ without the disease, and were 1.4 times more likely to have a diagnosis of gastro-oesophageal reflux disease.

They also compared medication use data for gastrointestinal disorders and endometriosis from the Australian Pharmaceutical Benefits Scheme (PBS) with the Australian Longitudinal Study on Women+'s Health (ALSWH), which provided further evidence of the likely co-occurrence of the diseases and disease symptoms.

What about adenomyosis?

You might have also heard the term 'adenomyosis' before. Approximately one-third of patients with endometriosis also have adenomyosis, which is a condition where endometrial-like tissue grows into the muscular wall of the uterus (myometrium). It is confined to the uterus, causing it to enlarge. This is more common in women+ in their forties and fifties who have given birth at least once, as well as those who have had uterine surgery.

Adenomyosis often causes heavy and painful periods and pelvic pressure. Both conditions can significantly impact quality of life and may require specialised care from a gynaecologist; for example, the presence of adenomyosis may make it harder to get pregnant and increase the risk of miscarriage.

Does endometriosis have different stages or levels?

Between 1973 and 2021, 22 endometriosis classification, staging and reporting systems were published, but there is still no international agreement on how to describe the disease. If the experts can't define endometriosis, how do they expect those living with it to express it in a way that is understood?

The most common classification is the Revised American Society of Reproductive Medicine (rASRM; American Society for Reproductive

Medicine; 1996), which was developed as a four-stage classification for endometriosis based on the endometrial lesions, specifically the number of endometrial implants and their depth.

Stage 1 is identified by minimal lesions, few superficial implants (they may be located on the ovarian peritoneum), and possibly the absence of symptoms, although some individuals may experience mild pelvic discomfort or painful periods (dysmenorrhea), occasional pain during intercourse (dyspareunia) and infertility.

Stage 2 presents as mild lesions, and painful periods may be more frequent, along with pelvic discomfort and a heightened risk of infertility due to pelvic adhesions. There may be more and deeper implants (which may be located on the ovarian peritoneum, the tissue that supports the ovaries and the fallopian tubes). Pelvic pain may be moderate, particularly during menstruation and ovulation. Pain during intercourse may also be more frequent.

Stage 3 involves moderate lesions, with many deep implants, small cysts on one or both ovaries, and filmy adhesions. Severe pelvic pain can be debilitating and impact daily activities. Chronic pelvic discomfort throughout the menstrual cycle is common. Other symptoms include persistent period pain and painful sex; gastrointestinal symptoms, such as bloating, constipation or diarrhoea; and an elevated risk of infertility due to compromised ovarian function and fallopian tube blockage close to the ovary (tubal occlusion).

Stage 4 is identified by many deeply implanted lesions, dense adhesions and large cysts on one or both ovaries. Excruciating pain is common, with extensive pelvic involvement leading to significant adhesions and organ dysfunction.

Severe menstrual cramps and painful sex, painful bowel movements and urination, heavy periods, and spotting or bleeding between periods can significantly impact quality of life and mental health.

Another staging classification system by the American Association of Gynecologic Laparoscopists (AAGL, 2021) was reviewed in Australia in 2024 but was found to be 'not superior' to the rASRM staging system.

The EndoFound Classification (2018) was developed by the Endometriosis Foundation of America. It proposed using more descriptive categories based on the anatomical location within the pelvis and the abdominal cavity and the level of infiltration. The EndoFound categories are:

- *Category I: peritoneal endometriosis:* The most minimal form of endometriosis, where the peritoneum (the membrane that lines the abdomen) is infiltrated with endometriosis tissue.
- *Category II: ovarian endometriomas (chocolate cysts):* Endometriosis is already established within the ovaries, but the chocolate cysts are at risk of breaking and spreading endometriosis into the pelvic cavity.
- *Category III: deep infiltrating endometriosis I (DIE I):* The first form of deep infiltrating endometriosis involves organs within the pelvic cavity, which can include the ovaries, rectum and the uterus, and can even lead to 'frozen pelvis' when the organs become attached together by scar tissue or adhesions.
- *Category IV: deep infiltrating endometriosis II (DIE II):* A more extreme form of deep infiltrating endometriosis involves organs both within and outside the pelvic cavity, including the bowel, appendix, diaphragm, heart, lungs and brain.

Your doctor might also mention three types of endometriosis, which are included in the ESHRE Information on Endometriosis based on the ESHRE Guideline on Endometriosis (Endometriosis guideline for patients, 2022).

- *Superficial peritoneal endometriosis:* The lesions involve the peritoneum and may be flat and shallow. They do not invade the space underlying the peritoneum. This is the most common form.
- *Cystic ovarian endometriosis (ovarian endometrioma):* An endometrioma is a cyst, usually found in the ovaries, in which the wall of the cyst contain endometriosis. The cysts are filled with old blood, which affects the colour, which is why they are also referred to as 'chocolate cysts'. Most women+ with endometrioma cysts will also have superficial and/or deep endometriosis present elsewhere in the pelvis. This form is less common.
- *Deep endometriosis:* Also known as DIE, an endometriosis lesion is defined as deep if it has invaded at least 5 millimetres beyond the surface of the peritoneum. Given the peritoneum is very thin, deep lesions always involve tissue underlying the peritoneum (the retroperitoneal space) or pelvic organs. This is the least common form.

Be aware

Stages don't predict the severity of pain. While the staging of endometriosis provides a framework for understanding the extent of the disease, the severity of pain experienced by individuals can vary widely and is influenced by factors beyond the stage alone.

Be prepared

Individuals found to have stage 1 (minimal), or stage 2 (mild) endometriosis may experience severe pain, while those with stages 3 and 4 may have few or no symptoms. The stage you are diagnosed with will not necessarily define or explain your levels of pain.

This can be challenging; you may feel like a bit of a 'fraud or a faker' finding out you have stage 1 endo if you report your pain as severe. You're not exaggerating; pain is as individual as you are.

Endo myths and facts

Unfortunately, there is so much misinformation and scuttlebutt out there about endometriosis, it can be really difficult to find a name for your pain and other symptoms—and Dr Google and social media don't provide evidence-based, medically sound information relevant to you. Your physical and mental health experience is unique and deserves to be seen, heard, diagnosed and treated. This book, the resources and the references provide trustworthy and relevant information. Let's 'endo' the confusion and clear the wood from the tri-osis.

Myth: Pregnancy cures endometriosis.

Fact: Pregnancy may lessen symptoms temporarily because, when pregnant, the menstrual cycle stops, and the estrogen doesn't signal the endometriosis tissues to grow and bleed. Once the normal monthly cycle returns after childbirth, leading to periods resuming, symptoms and lesions often return.

Myth: Severe period pain is normal.

Fact: Severe period pain that interferes with daily life is not normal and should be investigated with a doctor.

Myth: Endometriosis is rare in teenagers and young women+.

Fact: Endometriosis can affect children from the age of eight, teenagers and young women+.

Myth: Hormonal treatments cure endometriosis.

Fact: Hormonal treatments only suppress symptoms temporarily. Surgery by a gynaecologist, preferably accredited by the Australasian Gynaecological Endoscopy and Surgery Society (AGES) is the only effective medical treatment for removing endometriosis lesions.

Myth: You can't get pregnant with endometriosis.

Fact: While endometriosis can cause infertility, 70 per cent of women+ with the condition are still able to conceive, either naturally or with fertility treatment. Early diagnosis and treatment can reduce the rates of infertility. Hormonal medicines have varying levels of contraception.

Myth: Hysterectomy cures endometriosis.

Fact: Removing the uterus does not cure endometriosis; it stops adenomyosis and heavy menstrual bleeding, and you will no longer have periods or be able to carry a baby. Endometriosis lesions similar to the lining of the uterus can continue to grow elsewhere in the body, mainly in the pelvic cavity.

Myth: Endometriosis is caused by emotional issues.

Fact: Endometriosis is a physiological disease with complex hereditary, epigenetic and molecular causes, not an emotional condition.

Myth: Abortion or douching causes endometriosis.

Fact: There is no scientific evidence linking douching (flushing the vagina with water) or abortion with the development of endometriosis.

Myth: Endometriosis can be diagnosed through blood or urine tests.

Fact: Endometriosis cannot be diagnosed via these tests; specialised imaging or laparoscopy is required. Research is underway to study the efficacy of pathology tests, but it has not been validated.

Myth: Endometriosis only affects women+.

Fact: Endometriosis affects people presumed female at birth based on sex characteristics. It can, therefore, affect transgender, non-binary and gender-diverse individuals. In this book, we refer to women+ to include all individuals designated female at birth, which may include transgender individuals.

For trustworthy, evidence-based information, visit EndoZone, Jean Hailes for Women's Health, Julia Argyrou Centre for Endometriosis at Epworth and other websites listed in the resources section.

What causes endometriosis?

So now that we know what endometriosis is (and isn't)...what actually causes it? Unfortunately, the exact cause of endometriosis is still unknown. Research on this is ongoing and there are a number of medical theories. Environmental factors are also thought to play a role, with some chemicals thought to interfere with the body's endocrine (hormone) system (endocrine disruptors).

What might be going on in the body?

Let's get a bit nerdy. Here are some technical terms you might have heard, or might want to know more about, relating to important theories about what causes endo in 14 per cent of girls and women+. There are more questions than answers, which is why research is so important, and you can help by taking part in studies. Here are some theories:

Estradiol

Estradiol is a form of estrogen, a hormone that plays a crucial role in the reproductive system. It determines how the tissue in the uterus grows and regulates the menstrual cycle. It also signals the endometriosis lesions to grow and this triggers inflammation that is linked to pain.

Retrograde menstruation

Backwards, or retrograde menstruation, occurs when menstrual blood flows backward through the fallopian tubes into the pelvic cavity instead of leaving the body. This can cause endometrial cells to implant and grow outside the uterus, contributing to endometriosis.

Endocrine disruptors

Epigenetics is the study of how our genes are impacted by the environment we live in; for example, what we eat and what chemicals we are exposed to, which can disrupt your hormones. 'Endocrine disruptors' are chemicals that can interfere with the endocrine (hormone) system in the body. Ultimately, they can cause changes in the way your body's cells perform. This is known as an 'epigenetic process', meaning it relates to your genes and the way your DNA turns your genetic code into functions—and one of the functions that can be disrupted is estrogen production. When it comes to endo in particular, it's suspected that endocrine disruptors might interfere with our steroidogenesis genes. These genes are crucial for the production of hormones like estrogen, and disruption can lead to abnormal growth of endometrial tissue outside the uterus, a characteristic of endometriosis.

Environmental factors can affect hormones

Endocrine disruptors can be naturally produced (like phytoestrogens in soy) or man-made (like industrial chemicals, pesticides, plastics and pharmaceuticals). Growing evidence and research show these disruptors impact endometriosis, which is influenced by estrogen. Endocrine disruptors that mimic or interfere with estrogen can potentially worsen the condition as they:

- mimic natural hormones: tricking the body into overreacting or reacting at the wrong time
- block hormones: preventing natural hormones from binding and functioning properly
- alter hormone levels: interfering with the production, transport and breakdown of hormones, leading to imbalances.

Those living with endometriosis can also have other health challenges, which we explore later, and the impacts of endocrine disruptors can include:

- reproductive issues: infertility, early puberty and developmental issues in foetuses
- metabolic disorders: obesity, diabetes and thyroid problems
- cancer: some are associated with an increased risk of cancers, particularly hormone-related cancers like breast and prostate cancer.

These chemicals are found in many everyday items, including food packaging, cosmetics, toys and household cleaners. Exposure can also occur through environmental contamination, as industrial processes and agricultural practices result in the presence of these disruptors in air, water and soil.

Women+ exposed to endocrine disruptors while in the womb may have a higher risk of developing endometriosis. These chemicals can interfere with hormone function and lead to changes in the developing foetus.

Be aware

You can reduce exposure to endocrine disruptors and chemicals by being mindful of your cleaning and gardening products and opting for safer alternatives when possible. Look for natural products, including cloths made from ecofriendly cotton, bamboo, hemp, linen and recycled fabric that can be washed. You can also make your own cleaners at home, which is much cheaper and healthier. Vinegar, baking soda, rubbing alcohol, dish soaps and citrus oils can reduce fumes and artificial smells. Take precautions with garden chemicals, use gloves, cover skin and wear a mask.

Be prepared

You may feel powerless to avoid endocrine disruptors, but you can choose to avoid plastic containers, bottles and packaging, canned food and beverages, fast and processed foods. Instead, choose fresh and organic food, and supplement your diet with vitamin C, iodine and folic acid.

You can't prevent endometriosis, but you can reduce its symptoms and impact by limiting exposure to chemicals; maintaining a healthy diet; avoiding alcohol, caffeine and soft drinks; exercising regularly; and aiming to have a low percentage of body fat.

This book aims to encompass up-to-date and clinically sound evidence-based information. Sections on diet (Chapter 10), exercise (Chapter 11) and self-care (Chapter 12) will empower you on your journey with endometriosis.

CHAPTER 2

Understanding the pain and fatigue

Understanding pelvic pain

Pain from endometriosis often doesn't match the extent of the disease. As discussed in Chapter 1, endometriosis can be categorised as stage 1 (mild endometriosis) to stage 4 (the most severe), but this does not automatically correlate to the levels or types of pain a person experiences. Instead, pain tends to be more related to where the endometriosis deposits are located and how deeply they penetrate.

The International Association for the Study of Pain defines pain as: 'Unpleasant sensory and emotional experience associated with or resembling that associated with actual or potential tissue damage.'

The European Association of Urology defines chronic pelvic pain syndrome as:

> *Persistent pain in structures related to the pelvis ... is often associated with negative cognitive, behavioural, sexual and emotional consequences, as well as with symptoms and signs related to the lower urinary tract, sexual, bowel, pelvic floor or gynaecological dysfunction.*

The aptly named *endo*cannabinoid (ECS) system affects pain, inflammation, mood, sleep, appetite and digestion, immune function, memory and learning. Studies have shown that in women+ with endometriosis, the ECS impacts inflammation, the growth of lesions and the perception of pain.

Endo warriors will relate to the term 'paingry' to describe the impact of pain on moods.

By definition, persistent pelvic pain is felt most days and lasts for more than six months. It is a complex chronic pain condition affecting the pelvic region, below the belly button and between the hips, where the bowel, bladder, ovaries, uterus and fallopian tubes are located. It is estimated to affect between 15 and 25 per cent of women+ of child-bearing age until menopause. It is believed that 50 to 60 per cent of women+ with chronic pelvic pain have endometriosis.

The *Pelvic Pain in Australian Women* report (2023) by Jean Hailes for Women's Health found that almost half of Australian women+ have experienced pelvic pain in the last five years, and 28 per cent of all Australian women+ reported difficulty performing daily activities due to pelvic pain.

It also found that 21 per cent of all Australian women+ needed to take leave or an extended break from exercise (48 per cent), work or study (45 per cent) because of pelvic pain. Mental and emotional wellbeing was reported as an issue for 27 per cent of all Australian women+; in comparison, 15 per cent said it hurt their relationship with a partner, and 31 per cent indicated their relationships with partners were negatively affected, while 22 per cent reported issues with friendships and family relationships.

Inflammation and nerves

Endometriosis does not just affect the reproductive organs but can also have broader impacts on the nervous system, contributing to the complex nature of the condition. The relationship between inflammation, nerve endings and pain signalling in endometriosis is important. Nerves allow communication between different parts of the body by sending sensory information from our skin, muscles and internal organs to the brain. This allows us to sense pain. Nerves also carry signals from the brain to muscles and glands, enabling voluntary movements (like walking) and involuntary actions (like heartbeat and digestion).

Pain in endometriosis is both inflammatory and nerve-related, which makes it harder to treat and means it may need different approaches.

Endometriosis also affects the autonomic nervous system, including the sympathetic (the signals that put you on alert) and parasympathetic (the signals that tell you to relax) components. Imbalances in this system contribute to the overall pain experience and other symptoms associated with the condition.

Understanding these interactions with the nervous system helps in developing better treatments for endometriosis pain. We need more research to learn how to target inflammation, nerve growth and pain sensitivity to provide better relief.

Endometriosis lesions have more nerves than healthy tissue, and these nerves are mostly sensory, which means they are more sensitive to pain. Inflammation in endometriosis helps nerves and blood vessels grow, with chemicals like prostaglandins and nerve growth factor also making the nerves grow and become more sensitive.

Constant inflammation makes pain-sensing nerves more sensitive, meaning they react more easily to pain and cause more pain sensitivity (hyperalgesia). Chronic pain can also make the central nervous system more sensitive, leading to more intense pain.

When we feel pain, memories are made in the brain; the next time we feel it, our body remembers it, intensifying the feeling. The growth of new nerves and blood vessels (neuroangiogenesis) makes the lesions even more pain-sensitive, triggering the pain response faster. This can lead to escalating pain, even if the initial cause (such as a lesion or inflammation) is treated or reduced.

Endo's impact on the brain

Neuroimaging studies show that endometriosis affects brain function, especially in areas related to pain, emotions and thinking. These changes may explain why people with endometriosis often experience chronic pain.

Magnetic resonance spectroscopy works like an MRI, providing a non-invasive 'window' to measure neurotransmitters. This imaging has shown how endometriosis affects the brain, especially in areas related to pain, emotions and thinking.

About 40 per cent of your brain is made up of 'grey' matter (the main neural cell bodies, dendrites that receive signals from other nerve cells and the synapses that connect them). Women+ with endometriosis often have less grey matter in the thalamus, the area that processes and transmits information from the senses like touch, pain, temperature and pressure (apart from smell), to the appropriate brain areas. Grey matter plays a role in regulating sleep; and involves the insula area that is involved in emotion, perception of pain, hunger and fatigue. These symptoms are more noticeable in women+ with chronic pelvic pain from endometriosis.

Endometriosis is also linked to higher rates of anxiety and depression. Studies have shown that endometriosis can lead to altered gene expression in areas like the amygdala and hippocampus, which are crucial for managing anxiety and emotional responses. This suggests that the chronic pain associated with endometriosis may not only affect physical health but also significantly impact mental wellbeing.

Memory and concentration can be impacted by chronic pain, exacerbating the challenges faced by those with endometriosis, and causing the brain fog reported by so many due to the activation of the pain pathways.

Other causes of abdominal and pelvic pain

We know how long the journey to endometriosis diagnosis can be. The following conditions can be experienced alongside endo, or lead to your endo symptoms being misdiagnosed. If in doubt, check it out with your GP.

Small intestinal bacterial overgrowth

Small intestinal bacterial overgrowth (SIBO) occurs when there is an abnormal increase in bacteria in the small intestine. This overgrowth can lead to fermentation of undigested food, producing gases such as hydrogen and methane, which contribute to symptoms like bloating, abdominal pain, and diarrhoea or constipation.

Women+ with endo often have impaired food movement through the digestive system. When nerves and muscles are not contracting or relaxing properly, sluggish movements occur. As a result, food can stay there longer, and the bacteria feast, grow and prosper. This can lead to a 'leaky gut', caused when the bacteria produce toxins that damage the intestinal lining allowing harmful substances that are

20 The Australian Guide to Living Well with Endometriosis

better in that out, leaking into the bloodstream. This condition can exacerbate inflammation and contribute to a range of symptoms that blend in with those caused by endometriosis, such as abdominal pain and bloating. SIBO can interfere with nutrient absorption, leading to deficiencies in essential vitamins and minerals, such as B12 and fat-soluble vitamins (A, D, E, K).

Managing SIBO through dietary changes may mean incorporating probiotic and prebiotic foods, such as yoghurt, kefir and fibre-rich vegetables, to support a healthy gut microbiome. A dietitian may guide you through short-term restrictive diets and long-term lifestyle modifications. See more about diet and supplements in Chapter 6.

Interstitial cystitis

Interstitial cystitis affects the bladder, with worsening pelvic pain in the lead-up to menstruation and particularly after sex, and also leads to pressure and a frequent, often urgent need to wee. Symptoms are similar to endometriosis, and it is not uncommon for women+ to have both. Some specific foods seem to set it off, and symptoms tend to improve when citrus fruits, tomatoes, chocolate, coffee and caffeinated drinks, alcohol, spicy foods and soft drink are eliminated.

Inflammatory bowel disease

Inflammatory bowel disease is a group of inflammatory conditions of the colon and small intestine. Crohn's disease and ulcerative colitis are the main ones, and a study published in 2023 found endometriosis was detected in two-thirds of inflammatory bowel disease patients with compatible symptoms.

Urinary tract infections

Urinary tract infections affect the urinary system, including the bladder, urethra and kidneys. According to Jean Hailes for Women's Health, one in two women+ will get a urinary tract infection in their lifetime, and about one in three women+ will have a urinary tract infection needing treatment before they are 24 years of age.

Mesenteric adenitis

Mesenteric adenitis often affects girls under 16 years of age. Inflammation of the mesenteric lymph nodes can cause abdominal pain, and is usually caused by a viral infection, such as gastroenteritis. Pain and tenderness are often accompanied by nausea and vomiting.

Pelvic inflammatory disease

Sexually transmissible infections, such as chlamydia, mycoplasma genitalium and gonorrhoea, are the most common causes of infection and inflammation of the female reproductive organs. Pelvic inflammatory disease can lead to scarring of the fallopian tubes and infertility if it is left untreated or you have repeated episodes. It can also cause significant pelvic pain.

Fibroids (myoma or leiomyoma)

Fibroids produce symptoms similar to those experienced with endometriosis, with long, painful or heavy periods. About 20 to 30 per cent of women+ experience symptoms related to fibroids, which are non-cancerous tumours of fibrous tissue that may occur in the uterine (womb) wall. It is estimated that 70 per cent of women+ aged under 50 have them. Fertility can be affected, and surgical myomectomy (to remove the tumours) or hysterectomy are sometimes required. After menopause, fibroids usually shrink and may disappear.

Polycystic ovarian syndrome (PCOS)

The most common hormonal disorder in women+ of reproductive age affects about one in ten women+, and symptoms include heavy, irregular or no periods. This syndrome also results in a higher risk of diabetes.

Fatigue or low energy

The chronic inflammation caused by endometriosis can result in persistent, even extreme, fatigue and lack of energy, even outside of menstrual periods.

The presence of endometrial-like tissue outside the uterus triggers an immune response, leading to the release of cytokines and other inflammatory markers. This chronic inflammation can result in significant fatigue as the body expends energy to combat the disease. Hormonal imbalances can also impact energy levels.

Chronic pelvic and other pain is exhausting, and fatigue associated with endometriosis can have a profound impact on various aspects of life, such as showering or preparing meals, unloading the dishwasher or getting the mail. Any activity can result in needing to lie down.

This fatigue is distinct from typical tiredness; it is exhaustion that is hard to describe and is debilitating—even simple tasks deplete your energy. Endometriosis affects performance and attendance, leading to challenges like difficulty in completing educational goals, maintaining employment, and this can result in financial distress. This fatigue can lead to social isolation because of the need to cancel plans due to tiredness and other symptoms like pain and heavy menstrual bleeding.

Myalgic encephalomyelitis (chronic fatigue syndrome)

Studies suggest having endometriosis increases the likelihood of having chronic fatigue syndrome (ME/CFS), a complex, multisystem neuroimmune condition classified as a neurological disorder in the World Health Organization's International Classification of Diseases. According to the latest research, the prevalence of ME/CFS in Australia is estimated to be between 0.4 and 1 per cent of the population, which translates to up to 250000 people living with the condition.

Like endometriosis, its causes are a mystery. It may be triggered by a combination of factors, including viral infections, immune system problems, genetics and stress.

Of course, chronic fatigue varies from person to person and can 'flare-up', just like endo does. Some individuals may experience periods of improvement followed by relapses, while others may have more consistent symptoms.

An exercise physiologist or other health professional may say to 'count the wins'. When doing small tasks that shouldn't sap your energy, celebrate them as achievements. We cover Spoon Theory in Chapter 12, which talks about knowing your limits, conserving your energy and feeling you have some control over the body you're so angry with, which will relax your brain enough to lower the alert responses. Give it a try. It works for me.

Anaemia

One of the primary reasons women+ with endometriosis develop anaemia is due to heavy menstrual bleeding. This excessive bleeding can deplete the body's iron stores, resulting in iron-deficiency anaemia. The inflammatory response in endometriosis can lead to changes in iron metabolism, reducing iron absorption in the intestines and affecting the body's ability to use it effectively.

Diagnosis of iron-deficiency anaemia typically involves blood tests to check haemoglobin levels and iron stores. For women+ with endometriosis, managing anaemia may include dietary changes to increase iron intake, especially if you are vegetarian, vegan, pescatarian or experiencing nausea. Eating iron-rich foods and vitamin C to enhance absorption is important. If iron supplements are needed, side effects, such as tummy upsets, cramps, diarrhoea and constipation, are common — so is black poo. While these are negative side effects, the effects of not taking the supplements is worse. As I still need to remind my adult daughters, supplements won't work if you don't take them!

Be aware

Fatigue is a common symptom of endometriosis. According to Australian research published in 2024, 90 per cent of those living with the condition experience fatigue. A Swiss study found that 50.7 per cent of women+ with endometriosis reported experiencing frequent fatigue, compared with only 22.4 per cent of study participants without the condition. It is thought that the signals we discussed on page 18, which cause inflammatory communication throughout the body, also play a role in causing fatigue.

Be prepared

Naturally, addressing the underlying cause of blood loss is vital to treating anaemia. This is an important reason for treating endometriosis: to reduce estrogen and minimise the symptoms, including heavy menstrual bleeding and tiredness.

Unwelcome friends

By now you may have had a lightbulb moment—my pain and lived experience are not normal.

You're not alone.

The largest study to date into the genetics of endometriosis has found genetic links with 11 other inflammatory and pain conditions. Many of these conditions affect women+ more than men. Gender lottery once again for all the wrong reasons.

Am I more likely to have other chronic conditions as well as endo?

Women+ with endometriosis are at higher risk of infertility; ovarian, endometrial and breast cancers; melanoma; asthma; and autoimmune and cardiovascular disease.

Ovarian cancer risk

According to a US study of nearly 500 000 women+ aged 18 to 55, those with endometriosis had a higher risk of developing ovarian cancer, compared to those without it. In Australia, we refer to the main stages of ovarian cancer as numbered 1 to 4, which I have used here; note that in the US, they use the term 'type'. The research study found that the risk to participants with endometriosis was about four times greater (4.20 times) for all types of ovarian cancer. The risk was even higher for stage 1 ovarian cancer, which was about 7.5 times greater.

The highest risk of ovarian cancer was found in women+ with severe forms of endometriosis, such as DIE or ovarian 'chocolate' cysts (endometriomas). For all ovarian cancers, the risk was nearly ten times greater (9.66 times), while for stage 1 ovarian cancer, it was almost 19 times greater (18.96 times). For stage 2 ovarian cancer, the risk was about 3.7 times greater.

Additional prevention studies are necessary to better determine the link between endometriosis and ovarian cancer. Women+ with endometriosis could be an important population for cancer screening for further research.

Understanding the pain and fatigue **25**

Types of ovarian cancer associated with endometriosis

Research has identified a strong link between endometriosis and certain subtypes of epithelial ovarian cancer (which makes up 85 to 90 per cent of ovarian/fallopian tube cancers), particularly:

- Clear cell carcinoma: Women+ with endometriosis have an approximately three times increased risk of developing clear cell ovarian carcinoma.
- Endometrioid carcinoma: The risk of developing endometrioid ovarian carcinoma is about two times higher in women+ with endometriosis.
- High-grade serous carcinoma: There is a less pronounced but still notable association with high-grade serous cell cancers.

Genetic and molecular links

Research by Dr Sally Mortlock at the University of Queensland highlights key genes and regions of DNA that could help us better understand the connection between endometriosis and ovarian cancer. By analysing large-scale genetic data for both, researchers found that they share significant genetic similarities. The level of genetic correlation varies among different types of ovarian cancer, indicating that different biological pathways might be involved.

While the increased risk of ovarian cancer in women+ with endometriosis is a concern, it remains relatively low. However, the association underscores the importance of vigilant monitoring and appropriate management of endometriosis. Early detection and treatment of endometriosis may help mitigate some of the associated risks, including the potential development of ovarian cancer.

Be prepared

Regular medical follow-ups and discussions with healthcare providers about the potential risks and symptoms of ovarian cancer are essential for early detection and management. Understanding the link between endometriosis and ovarian cancer can lead to better screening strategies and potentially life-saving interventions for those at higher risk. See the resources for symptoms and signs.

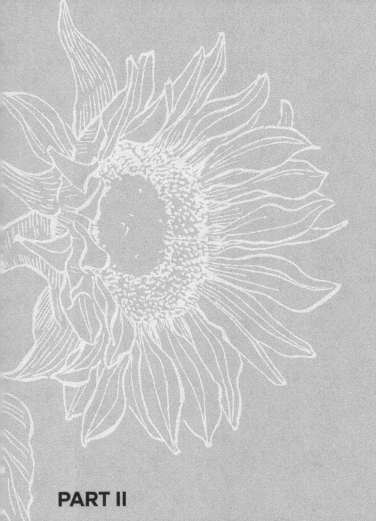

PART II
Track, Tell, Test
Getting a diagnosis

CHAPTER 3

How do I find a name for my pain?

Endo is more common than you think

We talked about symptoms in Chapter 1, so you know what is not normal—and it's important to know that doesn't mean *you're* not normal. You didn't choose endo; endo chose you.

With so many symptoms, you've probably been confused about what is normal. There's no point beating yourself up about delaying a visit to the GP or waiting to get checked out. As females, we are conditioned to think period and other pain is normal, to 'suck it up, princess'. Awareness through information and education has improved since 2018, particularly with the Australian NAPE and media campaigns with endo warriors empowered to share their lived experiences.

However, symptoms are normalised when the women+ around us have the same issues. You'll read accounts from our storytellers about mums, aunts and grandmothers who probably had endo and weren't diagnosed. In addition to the pelvic pain and heavy menstrual bleeding, other symptoms (such as experienced with IBS and SIBO, see page 20) can also hide endometriosis.

According to news.com.au's endo warrior and journalist Lexie Cartwright (who designed the campaign with me and was the face of it), the About Bloody Time survey of more than 1700 Australian women+ found that 54.4 per cent of those living with endometriosis were dismissed by their health practitioner when they sought help with their symptoms. It also revealed that only 32 per cent were diagnosed within six years, 45 per cent waited even longer than the average 6.5 years, while 22.4 per cent were still waiting for a formal diagnosis.

The journey to get tested and diagnosed

Now you need to get a name for your pain and start treating it. Full stop. Period. The risks of complications and infertility are too great to wait.

As we embark on our journey through the medical world, you'll learn about the four Ds doctors use, which we mentioned earlier:

- *dysmenorrhoea:* painful periods with cramping or pain 'below the belt' in the lower abdomen during the menstrual cycle
- *dyspareunia:* difficult, painful sex
- *dyschezia:* poo problems, trouble passing stools or loose bowel movements
- *dysuria:* pain or discomfort when urinating.

Throughout this book you'll hear our storytellers recount the number of times they were dismissed, disbelieved and had their pain discounted. They were gaslit, another word you need to learn, meaning health providers, parents and teachers made them feel their pain wasn't valid.

You may be made to feel that you are remembering things wrong or misinterpreting what you feel, both physically and mentally. Chances are, by the time you've booked an appointment with a GP, your symptoms have subsided, and you feel like a bit of a fraud, taking up the time of a busy doctor and wasting money and your time off. Wrong. We women+ are conditioned not to make a fuss and minimise pain, but that does not mean your pain is not valid.

This is compounded when GPs and health professionals lack an understanding of endometriosis, and they have little incentive or motive to upskill in pelvic pain, menstrual bleeding and general women+'s health.

If a health practitioner dismisses your symptoms, invalidates or trivialises your experiences, blames or shames you, ignores your medical history, or refuses to refer you for testing or to a specialist, get

30 The Australian Guide to Living Well with Endometriosis

a second or third opinion until you are taken as seriously as the pain you feel. To avoid the red flags, look for GPs specialising in women+'s health or visit federally funded endometriosis and pelvic pain clinics. More on this in the resources section.

You deserve a good quality of life and the opportunity to have children should you choose to. Don't wait, don't hesitate—seek a diagnosis and start your treatment journey to recovery.

Track your symptom impact

The best way to convey *all* your symptoms to health practitioners, not just the ones 'below the belt', is to show them a pattern over at least one month, but ideally many months or menstrual cycles. A recent study by Mitchell et al. aptly called 'The "most bothersome symptom" construct', asked participants to rate the impact of their symptoms on their lives. In order, they were:

- fatigue
- mood changes
- bloating
- period pain
- diarrhoea
- pelvic pain
- pain with bowel motions
- mid-menstrual cycle pain or pain around the time of ovulation
- nausea
- infertility
- pain with sexual activity
- constipation
- heavy menstrual bleeding
- bleeding between periods
- pain with urination
- vomiting
- general pain.

Those living with endometriosis, long derided and dismissed with inferences of emotional instability and hysteria, don't feel the term 'bothersome' does justice to their severe, debilitating and life-defining symptoms.

The study recommends instead asking the individual living with the pelvic pain to identify symptom impact and recommends a new measure to get to the bottom of what impacts them the most as well as supporting the use of the Endometriosis Impact Scale, The Endometriosis Impact Questionnaire and the Pelvic Pain Impact Questionnaire.

Raising Awareness Tool for Endometriosis

The Raising Awareness Tool for Endometriosis (RATE) was developed by gynaecologists, GPs, pain medicine specialists, fertility specialists, emergency physicians and nurses working with the Royal Australian and New Zealand College of Obstetricians and Gynaecologists (RANZCOG).

This tool (see the resources section for more) is recommended by gynaecologists and GPs and helps you to tell them what they need to know. When you complete it online, you're also helping to evaluate and improve the RATE and assist those living with endometriosis in describing and tracking their symptoms in a way that helps their GP or primary health provider identify and discuss symptoms that may be associated with endometriosis.

It is recommended that you complete the RATE and bring it with you when you visit your GP so they can include the information in the referral to a gynaecologist. Print it out or email it to your health practitioner to add to your medical file.

A long road to diagnosis: Jo's story

Dr Jo Armstrong is an endo warrior, and has earned a doctorate in business leadership, specialising in not-for-profit organisations. She is currently the CEO of Cystic Fibrosis Australia. Thanks to the work of Jo, other advocates, and especially the parents of those with cystic fibrosis, the life expectancy of this cohort has risen dramatically, with many people with cystic fibrosis living into their 40s, 50s and beyond.

Jo had been experiencing 'constant monthly pain' that was 'sometimes completely agonising and debilitating' since she was 13 years old. However, it wasn't until she was 41 that she was diagnosed with stage 3 endometriosis after undergoing laparoscopy surgery. Jo recalls her shock upon receiving the diagnosis and reflects on how she had normalised the pain for years, thinking, 'That's just what it's meant to be like'.

Her mother believed that 'really bad painful periods were a sign of high fertility', which added to the misconception that the pain she felt was normal. When Jo did mention her symptoms to doctors, she was often told it was normal or that surgery should only be considered if she wanted children. Reflecting on her younger self, Jo's words of advice are: 'This is not normal ... keep pushing to get a diagnosis.'

Jo emphasises the need for better awareness among healthcare providers about endometriosis, suggesting that a tool to track symptoms would have been helpful for her. She also highlights the importance of empowering women+ to recognise when their symptoms aren't normal and to seek appropriate care.

The struggle to be heard: Annastacia's story

Former Queensland Premier Annastacia Palaszczuk is an endo warrior. She was elected to parliament in 2006, and became leader of the opposition in 2012, premier in 2015 and retired from politics in 2023.

She has spoken openly of her endometriosis journey in the hope that she can raise awareness and encourage others to see their GP to discuss heavy periods and pain. Unfortunately, she thought painful cramps, pain when walking, exhaustion and headaches were normal. Her symptoms escalated when she was in her early thirties.

Sadly, she experienced a miscarriage and described the pain to her doctor, saying that the symptoms were like her 'normal' period. That prompted a referral to a specialist. Laparoscopic surgery found extensive endometriosis around her bowel and under her lungs. She had the surgery on the Friday and returned to work on the Monday, but urges women+ to take more time to recover instead of 'ploughing on'.

Unfortunately, despite four rounds of in vitro fertilisation (IVF), Annastacia discovered the extent of the endometriosis too late and was unable to have children. She was, however, able to help her younger sister when she experienced similar symptoms, and her endometriosis treatment at a younger age probably contributed to her different outcome—Annastacia's sister has two children now.

Annastacia believes social change is needed to stop pain from being normalised and urges openness in discussing symptoms relating to pelvic pain and visiting the GP with any concerns.

Be aware

You will find some tracking lists in the references. There's no need to pay for a period or fertility app, you can use your phone diary, notes or OneNote, which you can then print or email to your medical team.

If you prefer to use an app, download the free QENDO app to your phone: it is endometriosis-specific, and you won't be bombarded with stuff you don't need that may be triggering, particularly if you are challenged by fertility.

Be prepared

Fill in a pelvic pain and another tracking form, such as RATE (see page 32). Take a photo of it so you always have it handy for doctors' and specialists' appointments. Always take previous test results and imaging with you to medical appointments—this saves you time and money redoing them and may lead to a faster diagnosis by the 'right' doctor.

Heavy menstrual bleeding

Heavy periods with floods and blood clots are a huge issue for around a quarter of menstruating women+. In Australia, it is seldom discussed due to its stigma, lack of understanding, and the normalisation of its symptoms. As a result, heavy bleeding is dismissed and underdiagnosed.

According to guru gynaecologist Dr Talat Uppal, a clinical senior lecturer in gynaecology at Macquarie University and founder of Bleed Better, 50 per cent of those living with endometriosis experience heavy bleeding, leading to anaemia and other health complications. Symptoms like weakness (59 per cent); bleeding-related discomfort (48 per cent); nocturnal disruptions (34 per cent); and compromised social, professional, athletic or sexual lives (30 per cent) are reported.

If you're curious whether your bleeding is 'normal', take the survey 'Know your flow', created by pharmaceutical company Bayer — it's in the resources section.

Be aware

Professor Luk Rombauts was head of Reproductive Medicine at Monash Medical Centre and adjunct clinical professor in the Department of Obstetrics and Gynaecology at Monash University. He says:

> Those with endometriosis can have heavy menstrual bleeding, and if they have adenomyosis, could have very, very heavy periods. So if you're flooding, [and] you think this is uncontrollable bleeding, that's a reason to go to the emergency department. If the pain is just intolerable, you are fainting, you are experiencing pain that you would rate nine or ten out of ten, and nothing seems to work, go to hospital. They have medications that can be used intravenously, which can give short relief.

He urges women+ to 'advocate for themselves in a way that a very busy emergency department team will take them seriously'.

Be prepared

Professor Rombauts recommends keeping a file with all your recent health information, a list of medications and everything else you're on, as well as basic health and health fund information, as well as your Medicare card.

He strongly suggests that if you've already seen a specialist, ask, where possible, for copies of the operation report and the images from laparoscopies:

Take lots of photos and copies of your ultrasound reports because, when you go in, the first inclination of the emergency physician will be, all right, we'll need to do all of these tests, like ultrasounds. That will delay treatment.

What it means to be an endo warrior: Helen's story

Helen Schiele is an endo warrior, and has been my friend for over 40 years. Yet, for decades, I never knew the challenges she faced with endometriosis and heavy menstrual bleeding, fertility and pain. She didn't talk about it. She soldiered on. Helen has a master of education and is finishing her doctorate in pedagogical pathways. She says:

When seeking a definition of the word 'warrior', phrases and words such as 'distinguished in fighting', 'brave', 'experienced in battle', 'a person who shows great vigour', 'courageous', 'one who can fight to protect themselves', 'confident', 'strong', 'disciplined', come to mind. I realised these descriptions could apply to me. Coming from a military family, I can now, at 55, confidently say I am an endo warrior, having battled this condition since I was 12.

Helen vividly remembers starting menstruation and being informed by her mother that this would be a monthly occurrence for the next 40 years. Each month, her cycle became heavier, more painful and debilitating.

> *It all started with my very first period when I was 12, and it just went downhill from there. Really heavy bleeding every month was just traumatic. It took me a good week to get over the period, and it just went on and on, and I was just told that that was normal. That it was perfectly normal for you to have heavy bleeding. You just were unlucky that you had a heavy bleed—that was it. No GP would take my complaints seriously. I wasn't heard; my voice wasn't listened to.*

At age 14, Helen sought help from their family doctor, who recommended going on the pill. This was in the 80s, and it was very taboo. Breaking the news to her mother led to tension. Even on the pill, Helen had heavy menstrual bleeding and pain.

> *It was brutal on the family as well because they were walking on eggshells around me, trying to be supportive but not understanding what I was going through. I was going through so many pads a day. I couldn't wear a tampon because the bleeds were so heavy. Finally, a GP listened and suspected I had endometriosis, which I'd never heard about.*

When referred to a female specialist, Helen hoped for kindness and comfort but instead endured her first dilation and curettage, which is a procedure to remove tissue from inside the uterus. She had laparoscopies, with the specialist eventually suggesting pregnancy as a solution. Unsatisfied, Helen found another specialist and tried acupuncture, which offered slight relief but no lasting solution. 'I finally went to a Chinese herbalist for support because Western medicine wasn't working. I'd walk around with a needle on top of my head rather than endure another operation.'

Helen faced the possibility of a full hysterectomy. She struggled with the reality that pregnancy was unlikely. In 1995, Helen miscarried at four months, not even knowing she was pregnant, which left her devastated. Further examination revealed she was still pregnant with a twin, and a new gynaecologist helped her carry the pregnancy to full term. This child gave Helen renewed strength and purpose.

Unfortunately, the endometriosis returned after the pregnancy: 'It was full on. I ended up having a Mirena [hormonal intrauterine device] put in, and that alleviated some of the symptoms, but I still have days where the pain is there.'

Under her gynaecologist's care, Helen found new ways to manage her condition. Despite enduring further dilation and curettage procedures — she's had about 25 — and other treatments, her confidence began to return. Over the years, her symptoms became more manageable, with the aid of medication and the support of a loving partner who helped her through the worst times.

She says she wants others:

... to be heard and valued for their feelings rather than being told to take a Nurofen, a Panadol or a Bex and have a good lie down and you'll be fine. To say this is a real condition, and these are the pathways you can go through.

I think the most important thing is just having a doctor believe that your symptoms are real. If you are not heard by a general practitioner, then I would recommend that you be referred to a good AGES-certified gynaecologist for surgery.

My journey with endo has been a battle of wills; one where I started to feel I had the determination not to let it beat me, to be free from the silence of what this condition is and can do ... Now we have a voice, a battle cry to say, 'I am an endo warrior, and I suffer with this condition, and I demand help'. We need to find a cure for this condition.

CHAPTER 4

What kind of doctor do you need?

In this chapter, we'll discuss some of the different medical practitioners who you might meet on your journey towards diagnosis and treatment. It is important you know 'who is who in the zoo' and what they do.

Remember, be prepared with information—no-one knows your symptoms and the impact on your life better than you. Think of your body as a company with departments and divisions. You are the CEO. Review the reports coming from different parts of your body. Be proactive in tracking the highs and lows and consider what triggered those results: symptoms. Take the time to evaluate, question, reassess and rebalance your inputs. Consider setting goals for outputs and start a plan to achieve them. Little changes can have big impacts.

Build a team to support you in managing your company with you at its centre. If anyone on your team isn't supporting you, advocate for yourself and, if required, move on with someone who shares your vision and strategic plan for better health.

GPs (local or family doctors) generally work in clinics with other health providers, including allied health and complementary care. GPs play a crucial role in diagnosis and coordination, ensuring that patients receive comprehensive treatment that addresses their physical and psychological pain.

As we've talked about in Chapter 2, those experiencing persistent pelvic pain often have overlapping conditions such as IBS, fibromyalgia, postural orthostatic tachycardia syndrome (POTS) and migraines, as well as psychological factors like anxiety and depression. As mentioned in Chapter 3, it is important to be prepared for your appointment, armed with enough information on your lived experience over a long period (pardon the pun).

Early intervention and a collaborative approach can significantly improve outcomes for women+ suffering from persistent pelvic pain. There are several reasons for chronic pain below the belt that lasts six months or longer, including:

- pelvic organ issues: conditions such as endometriosis, adenomyosis, and fibroids
- musculoskeletal pain: issues involving pelvic floor muscles or other musculoskeletal structures
- central sensitisation: heightened sensitivity in the nervous system, making you more susceptible to pain.

GPs are often the first to discuss endometriosis and other potential reasons for your pain with you. They will ask what medications, if any, you're taking from the chemist 'over the counter' to manage your pain, and about any side effects from the medication. If your current medications aren't working, they may suggest a hormonal treatment.

If you have heavy menstrual bleeding or issues with peeing, your GP might want to check for anaemia and urinary tract infection. GPs can diagnose and treat illnesses, order blood and urine tests and, if needed, arrange infusions like iron and vitamins.

They can refer you for scans, such as x-rays as well as ultrasounds, which use soundwaves to diagnose ovarian cysts, fibroids and other conditions. Ultrasounds can usually see endometriosis on the ovaries or deep (DIE) (see page 10), although superficial endometriosis is hard to detect. Ultrasound isn't as invasive as surgery, but it is uncomfortable as it is done through the abdominal wall (transabdominal), through the vagina (transvaginal) or the rectum (transrectal). The latter two options involve a device being inserted and moved around.

What symptoms do GPs look for in endometriosis?

Endometriosis is sneaky, stealthy and, as we've talked about, can be masked by other conditions and symptoms. The Royal Australian College of General Practitioners (RACGP) conducted a review of recent evidence and guidelines, and offered some guidance on how to better detect endometriosis. It advises GPs to consider endometriosis when a woman+ reports one or more of the following symptoms, so make sure you keep a record of those D words and other symptoms, including:

- dysmenorrhoea (painful menstruation/period)
- deep dyspareunia (painful sex)
- dysuria (painful urination/pee)
- dyschezia (painful bowel movements/poo)
- haematuria (blood in urine)
- shoulder tip pain
- catamenial pneumothorax, (trouble breathing, pain in the shoulder blades, usually within 72 hours before or after onset menstruation)
- cyclical cough/haemoptysis (blood in your saliva from lungs or airways)/chest pain
- cyclical scar swelling and pain
- fatigue
- infertility.

Record your story. How old were you when the symptoms started? Has it changed? Is the bleeding heavier? Is the pain sharper, burning, always there, dull? How long have you been trying to get pregnant?

If you are concerned about getting pregnant, have experienced miscarriage or are interested in learning more about fertility preservation, they may refer you to a fertility specialist or public health clinic.

GPs act as coordinators, ensuring that all healthcare providers involved in the patient's care are informed and working together. This helps to avoid fragmented care and ensures that all aspects of the patient's condition are addressed.

Creating your care team and plan

Your GP can help coordinate your person-centred care, ensure you're not wasting time repeating the basics, and will keep an up-to-date record of all of your health information and treatment goals.

To help manage your symptoms holistically and more naturally, GPs coordinate multidisciplinary care. They might refer you to a pelvic physiotherapist, osteopath, acupuncturist, dietitian or psychologist.

(Some of these can be expensive unless provided as part of a treatment plan or through a federally funded endometriosis and pelvic pain clinic. You can find one close to you in our references section or Google it.)

For example, you need a referral to a gynaecologist or other specialist to receive the Medicare rebate. A referral letter includes your age, symptoms, medical history, medications and relevant information. A referral from a GP is valid for 12 months from the date of your first appointment or three months if another specialist or consulting physician writes it. A referral improves a specialist's ability to communicate and liaise with your GP for a treatment plan and follow-up.

If you're unhappy with a specialist or would like a second opinion, you can ask your GP for a referral to another specialist. You can often make this request without seeing the GP again; they can bulk-bill the time.

Chronic care plan services use any or all of the following.

General practitioner management plan

A general practitioner management plan focuses on your healthcare needs, health problems and relevant conditions. Your GP will record the management goals and actions needed, as well as the treatment and services you will need—and they will make arrangements or provide referrals for those treatments and services. An important part of this is a periodic review of the plan and how it is working.

Team care arrangements

Team care arrangements (essentially coordinated care between health practitioners) are made by the multidisciplinary team who will provide the treatments and services recommended by your GP.

GP mental health treatment plan

A mental health treatment plan lets you claim up to 10 individual and 10 group sessions with a mental health professional each calendar year, according to Services Australia. Given the impact endometriosis has on every aspect of a person's life, the ability to deal with the psychological and mental health and wellbeing effects of the disease are as important as the physical. A mental health treatment plan looks at the steps needed and the team who will provide the care. It outlines the steps you need to take to support yourself through the plan and will also embed times where the plan should be reviewed.

Getting a diagnosis when endo runs in the family: Ellie's story

Ellie Angel-Mobbs is one of Australia's top female radio presenters, and her trophy cabinet backs this up. With two decades of radio experience behind her, she has been a finalist for the Australian Commercial Radio Awards many times and was crowned Australia's best entertainment personality in 2022 and 2023.

Here she shares her journey and genes.

I'm really lucky. My mum is a huge role model, and I'm blessed to have someone like her by my side. So shout out to Barb. She is an absolute queen. We knew what endometriosis was because there was a history with her and her sisters. That helped in finding a 'name for my pain'.

I remember having a chat with my mum before I got my period. It was one of those awkward ones where as soon as they start talking about periods and, you know, sex ed and all that, you get all uncomfortable, and I tuned out. Still, I do remember hearing some words about endometriosis ...

When I did get my period, Mum just knew because I was unwell. I kept going to her and asking for Panadol. Of course, we monitored it, but I am lucky we had that family history. Mum had bad periods and chocolate cysts, my aunties had endometriosis, and one of my aunties had adenomyosis as well. Probably my Nana did, too. There's that strong hereditary link there; our family already had endo education.

My first period went for, like, two weeks, and it was really heavy. I remember one day, I had to tie my jumper around the back of my waist because I had bled through, and it was just awful and never really got any easier for me.

From the age of 16, my periods were all out of whack as well. I had them for two weeks, and then it wouldn't come for three months, and there was no regularity for me. So I went to the GP, I would have been around about 17, and Mum sat in there with me. The doctor just said we will put you on the oral contraceptive pill.

I remember the pill made me feel awful, and I gained weight. It was just this horrible, horrible time for me. I played competitive sports, too... I still get nervous about putting on any weight because of what happened to me in those formative years.

When I had my first laparoscopy surgery, they found endometriosis lesions on my bladder and bowel. In my most recent scan, it looked like the pouch of Douglas [at the back of the uterus] was fused to my bowel. But then I've also got lymphocytic colitis [affecting the large intestine], which they diagnosed from colonoscopies. Going to the toilet was horrific. I had a second laparoscopy and have lost count of how many other surgeries; I think it's about 20 due to endo complications.

Professor Danielle Mazza AM on how a GP diagnoses endo

Professor Danielle Mazza AM is a general practitioner and an absolute rockstar in the women+'s health sector. In 2023, she was awarded an Order of Australia for contributions to medical research, medicine and women+'s health, and received a fellowship from the Australian Academy of Health and Medical Sciences.

I was honoured to serve with her on the federal government Endometriosis Expert Advisory Group and the steering committee for Endo-MP. She's a leading advocate for evidence-based care and a vocal advocate for gender equity in medicine and health.

Professor Mazza is working with her team at Monash University's Sphere on the development of the first national Endometriosis Management Plan for GPs, funded under NAPE. It is an opportunity for systemic change.

Professor Mazza is very focused on GPs taking a comprehensive history, and trying to understand the nature of the pain, its location and its effect on women+'s lives.

We gather a picture of the most common scenarios or diagnoses through that information. If we're talking about pelvic pain, we need to consider everything in the pelvis, from the intestinal to the urinary to the reproductive systems. We also need to consider the patient's context and how the pain affects her work and study life.

I want to hear about the duration and timing of the pain. Do you have this pain every day? Are there periods of time when you don't have any pain? Does the pain wake you at night? Is the pain only when you exercise or is it only when you have sex? I learn and can understand its nature, frequency, persistence and the things that bring on the pain and relieve it. When you can understand the features and the timing, you get a better indication of its causation and can direct your investigation for your management accordingly.

There are also a number of tests to rule out causes.

Diagnostics is a puzzle. We need to differentiate between irritants to the bowel outside of the bowel, such as endometriosis, and inflammation in the intestine itself, which is more likely to be inflammatory bowel disease...

She stresses that treatment of endometriosis and other symptoms:

... are not going to turn around in one or two weeks; we need to give treatments a good go. If things were not settling, the next step would be a referral for medical imaging. Then, you'll probably be referring to a gynaecological service of some kind... I think women's health physios have a very strong role, and the guidelines recommend them in situations where the pain is chronic to help women with strategies to manage chronic pain and turn that around.

RACGP defines chronic conditions as present for six months or more.

Referral is not necessarily something that I would do in that first three to six months in the diagnostic process. The same goes for a dietitian. These are helpful after diagnosis where we're starting to get some chronicity in pain and in developing a kind of whole-person management strategy to manage this chronic condition.

Discussing the role of gynaecologists and GPs, she says:

My specialist colleagues are very good at investigating, confirming diagnoses and creating a management plan, but then they should encourage the patient to come back to the GP because a patient is more than just their endometriosis. They are whole people with health needs across a wide range of body systems and require attention for physical and mental health. A GP is a holistic practitioner. I think specialists can make recommendations and perform surgery where appropriate, and then the GP coordinates the care across various providers, including allied health.

For many women+ with endometriosis, fertility can be challenging due to the effect the condition has on a woman+'s body.

Endometriosis and fertility are closely entwined, but this also necessitates a careful and sensitive approach to conversations. What was once considered sound advice to women with endometriosis may not take into account the many factors that affect these decisions, such as the desire to have a child, stage of life, and financial and emotional stability.

Sometimes, the medical advice to young women with endometriosis is to 'have your children early, get pregnant as soon you can if you want a baby', and I understand it would be perceived as very stigmatising, demeaning and condescending if it's not understood correctly. So I think it's necessary to have a very delicate conversation delivered carefully.

Again, it is an issue around communication how the conversation goes and the nuance in that discussion. I wish we could have a fertility discussion with all women about what their reproductive goals are and how to achieve them best because, whether a woman has endometriosis or not, she needs to be aware of a range of things that she might not be happy to hear about. And I think, in general, young women don't have a good understanding about the consequences of age on fertility, the consequences of chronic disease on fertility, the consequences of endometriosis on fertility.

46 The Australian Guide to Living Well with Endometriosis

Be aware

You should check if your GP clinic bulk-bills and, if not, what the gap is between what Medicare covers and their fee. Ensure you get a copy of all reports (blood, urine etc.), and the GP adds it to your My Health Record (digitalhealth.gov.au) and sends it to everyone in your multidisciplinary team.

Be prepared

When visiting your GP or other health professional, have your Medicare card with you or at least the number, expiry date and the number next to your name if you share the card with others. If you have private health insurance or a concession card, take the details with you to get any rebates or cheaper services you're entitled to.

Be aware

GPs often prescribe the oral contraceptive pill, which is a medicine that is not just used for birth control. It can be an effective treatment for endometriosis and, while it cannot cure the condition, it can prevent the growth of new lesions, provide pain relief, regulate the menstrual cycle and even stop the cycle.

A referral to the gynaecologist

Medical doctors train an additional six years to become specialised in women+'s health care. Some of the roles they undertake include gynaecologists (focusing on the reproductive organs), obstetricians (specialising in the care of pregnant women+), and birth and fertility specialists working in assisted reproductive technology, including IVF.

Gynaecologists diagnose and treat persistent pelvic pain, endometriosis, adenomyosis, fibroids, heavy menstrual bleeding, ovarian cysts, cervical issues, infertility and pregnancy loss. They can offer medical, hormonal and surgical treatments as well as referrals to other specialists for multidisciplinary care.

Usually, there will be a physical examination, both outside and internally, through the vagina or rectum, or both. Be prepared with comfortable clothing and some period undies or pads just in case. If you have your period or bleeding, don't cancel; you're seeing an expert who's used to this. Sometimes it even helps them understand what's going on.

Dr Tarana Lucky on what to expect at the gyno

Lucky by name ... her patients are lucky to have her.

Dr Tarana Lucky is a qualified robotic advanced laparoscopic and minimally invasive gynaecologist based in Melbourne. She works at the Royal Women's Hospital and Epworth Hospital, and is a senior lecturer at the University of Melbourne.

When asked what patients should expect at the first appointment, she said:

> *I always start my assessment well before I see the patient. Whenever I see a referral for any type of pelvic pain or symptoms that may be consistent with endometriosis, I'll send the patient some questionnaires on quality of life and pelvic pain.*
>
> *I also send them a central sensitisation inventory questionnaire. This gives me a picture or landscape of where they are at the baseline even before I see the patient ... so that when I see them on-site in my rooms, I can focus and target those areas a bit more.*

Dr Lucky suggests that if you don't receive forms to complete from your gynaecologist before your appointment, you track your own symptoms so the medical practitioner can see the trend, as we outlined earlier.

> *I think one of the simplest ways to do it is to put it onto your phone calendar sometimes, your painful days. When does the pain arrive around your period? The days that you are taking time off because*

of pain. I encourage you to mark your pain scores out of ten on those days as well. Also, note when you take medications and pain relief.

She notes the:

... diverse range of symptoms that endometriosis can give you, and so many different types of pain. As a gynaecologist, I want to get to the bottom of your pain, starting with whether the period pain or pelvic pain is cyclical versus non-cyclical. I want to know if you have dysmenorrhoea (excessive pain during your period), dysuria (pain during urination), or dyschezia (trouble with bowel movements), dyspareunia (pain during sex).

Phew! We went through these four Ds earlier! The doctor will usually be just as comfortable with you talking about pain during or around your period, when you pee, poo and when you have sex. Don't be shy talking about which positions or actions hurt—it helps them understand your symptoms.

Be aware

As a result of the About Bloody Time campaign by news.com.au, which I am proud to be involved with, you are eligible for a longer gynaecologist specialist consultation of around endometriosis of 45 minutes or more, which is covered under Medicare from 1 July 2025.

Sometimes, when you book a specialist appointment, you may be asked for a copy of the referral to be sent to them before your consultation. Others may tell you to bring the letter with you on the day. You may be sent some forms or questionnaires to fill out, perhaps online, before the appointment.

Having to recount your lived experience with persistent pelvic pain, heavy menstrual bleeding, painful sex, toileting issues and fertility fears can be very emotional.

Gynaecologists, have studied for many extra years to gain knowledge and are keen to keep up to date through their peak body, RANZCOG. Those treating endometriosis and other problematic conditions are sympathetic to your pain. They specialise in women+'s health because they care deeply about it. If you don't 'click' with the specialist you've been referred to, ask to see another one or two. Make the most of your appointment time by being prepared in information, your tracked symptoms and pain experience, along with test results, medications and treatments you have tried, any side effects and family history, if relevant.

CHAPTER 5

What to expect from examinations and tests

To get a 'name for your pain', there's no blood, urine or menstrual blood test—you need a physical examination to rule out some reasons for your symptoms and to identify those that may be endometriosis. You may also need surgery—more about that in Chapter 7.

Diagnosing endometriosis involves assessing the symptoms you've tracked, describing your pain and discomfort, and undergoing a few tests, such as:

- clinical examination: a doctor does an internal examination and checks for any physical abnormalities
- medical imaging: ultrasound uses soundwaves to create pictures of the inside of your body
- laparoscopy: a minor surgery to examine the area internally (more on this in Chapter 7), where a thin telescope is inserted through a small cut in your abdomen to look inside. If endometriosis is suspected, tissue samples are taken for confirmation.

If you've lived with pain for a long time, you're not just physically hypersensitive; you may be emotionally fearful of being touched. This is called haphephobia, and this can cause you to feel anxious, panicky, nauseous and faint if you need to be examined, particularly around the abdomen, pelvic area, vulva (outside), vagina (inside) and rectum (backside). You may also be living with past physical and sexual trauma and being touched 'below the belt' may be triggering.

In the previous chapter, we looked at the kinds of medical professionals you may need to help diagnose and manage your endometriosis. In this chapter, we'll look a bit closer at some of the common procedures your doctor may recommend.

Rachel Andrew on preparing for a physical exam

Intimate examinations are sometimes a necessary part of women+'s health care to feel the movement and position of organs for medical diagnosis, pelvic floor physiotherapy, PAP smears and pelvic scans.

Rachel Andrew is a co-founder of Vagenius in Tasmania, which is approved as a national training provider for doctors at the RANZCOG, RACGP, and Australian College of Rural and Remote Medicine (ACRRM) and is evidence-based for EndoZone. She advises that, if you're nervous about the physical exam, there are exercises that can help you prepare at home before your medical appointment. By following these steps, you'll gradually get your body used to the physical sensations of intimate examination, and you'll be familiar with your stress cues and be able to help these feelings pass.

Go with how you are feeling on the day—move up and down the following levels described next as you need to. If you start to feel odd, shaky or cold, stay with the exercise and do deep abdominal breathing for a few seconds. If the feeling doesn't pass, stop for today and try again tomorrow. Aim to feel relaxed and comfortable at each level for two to three minutes.

- Level 1: Lie on your back, completely clothed, with a towel over your hips and pillows on the sides of your knees for support. Open your legs and rest your knees on the pillows.
- Level 2: Lie on your back, underpants on, all other clothes off, towel over your hips, legs closed.
- Level 3: Lie on your back, underpants on, all other clothes off, towel over your hips, legs open and rest your knees on the pillows.
- Level 4: Lie on your back, no clothes on, towel over your hips, legs closed.
- Level 5: Lie on your back, no clothes on, towel over your hips, legs open and relaxed, with your knees supported by pillows.

Notice any stressful sensations and then breathe until they pass. You'll be reassuring your body that you're in charge and safe.

At your appointment with the health practitioner, let them know if you're anxious and may need to stop for a breath. Know that the panicky feeling will pass and that you can stop anytime. Remember why you are there—to find the reasons for your pain and symptoms impacting your life.

Pelvic examination

It is empowering to be prepared, emotionally and physically, for a confronting physical examination by health practitioners. Many people find that when they understand what is going to happen and why, they feel less anxious. Professor Jason Abbott and Dr Supruni Kapurubandara developed *A GP Guide to Persistent Pelvic Pain* (2024), and Jason has helped me summarise the key points of what to expect during an examination. A pelvic examination will begin with the following steps:

- Starting position: The patient sits in a chair with both feet on the ground.
- Checking the lower back joints: The doctor feels each side of the lower back.
- Changing positions: The patient lies on their back with their knees bent and hips in a straight position.
- Hip muscle check: The doctor touches near the front of the hip bone to check the muscle.
- Stomach muscle check: The doctor touches the top part of the lower belly, near the pubic bone.
- Testing for pain: The doctor presses on the inside of the thigh to familiarise the patient with the examination process and provide a scale of reference for pain reporting. If tenderness is present at the inner thigh, this may indicate pelvic pain hypersensitivity/ central sensitisation.

Following these initial steps, the doctor will use one finger to feel the muscles inside your vagina in a circle-like motion. It usually starts on the right side, feeling the first muscle, then moves to the next muscle on the right. Before it switches to the left side, feeling the two muscles on that side.

What to expect from examinations and tests **53**

The doctor presses on each muscle and asks the patient to rate their pain with a number. For one of the muscles, you may be asked to push your leg outward while the doctor presses on it.

Medical imaging

An MRI is a painless procedure that produces detailed pictures without the use of x-ray radiation. It isn't recommended as a first scan because it is expensive; however, it can very accurately find endometriosis plaque formation, endometriosis on the ovaries or the bowel, extensive pelvic scarring, and abnormal fallopian tubes.

The RANZCOG recommends MRI for surgical planning when deep infiltrating endometriosis of the bowel, ureter or bladder is suspected. It helps health professionals plan pathways and also determine whether they need another specialist, such as a colorectal surgeon, if the endometriosis is impacting the intestines, bowel, or rectum.

Be aware

You are eligible for an MRI Medicare rebate (Item 63563) for fertility investigation or surgical planning for a patient with known or suspected deep endometriosis involving the bowel, bladder or ureter (or any combination), where the results of pelvic ultrasound are inconclusive. Ask for the referral to include this number.

Be prepared

You can only receive the rebate once every two years. You may be out of pocket unless the service is bulk-billed, and there are incentives for this. Out-of-hospital services attract higher benefits when they are bulk-billed by the provider.

Ultrasound

Ultrasound is a game changer for diagnosing endometriosis and also serves as a map for those who need a laparoscopic operation to treat it. It looks at seven 'markers' and shows the natural movement of the organs and highlights adhesions or scar tissue.

The RANZCOG recommends clinical (vaginal) examination and ultrasound imaging (urinary tract, digestive tract) based on signs and symptoms of endometriosis. Ultrasound can be used to detect endometriotic cysts or nodules on the bowel. Transvaginal ultrasound (TVUS) can also be used to diagnose DIE.

Imagendo

Using multimodal artificial intelligence methods, the Imagendo project, led by The University of Adelaide, is developing an accessible, cost-effective, non-invasive diagnostic tool for endometriosis. It can use information from MRIs and ultrasound scans to identify lesions and better plan surgery to treat endometriosis. More on this in the resources.

Be aware

An abdominal ultrasound is performed externally, and the sonographer will put some gel (hopefully warm) on the device and move it around your belly area. This is usually effective in finding issues with your ovaries and your uterus.

An internal ultrasound involves penetration of your vagina (transvaginal) or rectum (transrectal). The imaging tool, called a transducer, is inserted to locate the source of your pelvic pain, checking for endometriosis, adenomyosis, ovarian cysts, fibroids, infections and other issues. Sometimes, you need to have a wee first; other times, you need a full bladder. Take a bottle of water with you, just in case! It's all over in about 30 minutes.

Be prepared

There is a Medicare rebate (Item 55736) for an ultrasound scan of the pelvis to look at the inside of the uterus if a previous ultrasound showed an abnormality in parts of the reproductive system (uterus or fallopian tube). Ask for the referral to include this number.

When testing helps to name the pain: Kristy's story

Kristy Penrose is an endo warrior. She has an MBA and has worked for world-leading consulting, insurance and pharmaceutical companies. Kristy shares her journey from the onset of endo symptoms to diagnosis, thanks to her persistence and resilience.

I first got my period at 13 and immediately started experiencing period pain and heavy bleeding. I needed to miss days of school, and sports carnivals left me in tears and petrified of going. I grew up in a household where my mum and sister hadn't had any issues with their periods, and it was a Catholic household, which meant talking about the pill was off-limits.

When I was 18, I finally went on the pill; however, I kept having bad reactions to it. I would throw up fairly regularly, and my health literacy was poor—I thought it may have been normal, but I wasn't entirely sure. I didn't realise that it meant it probably wasn't working. All the doctors I had seen said there was nothing wrong.

At 20, I had an ectopic pregnancy. I woke in the middle of the night in excruciating pain and spent all night in tears; then, in the morning, I went to a doctor who sent me straight to the hospital and I had emergency surgery.

I was told at that time that my left fallopian tube wasn't working and that it was scarred. The doctor left it in and said that one day I might need to have it removed. He said this would not affect my ability to get pregnant. No-one mentioned endo/adenomyosis or anything like that.

I also asked about freezing my eggs. I was turned away many times, told I was too young to worry about that, and that the pain was all in my head. Something was nagging in my mind, but I didn't listen to it, I just pushed on. I went about my business, my periods got heavier, my pain developed more 'out of cycle', and I started developing bowel and bladder issues, as well as anxiety. Anxiety about leaving the house, playing sport, going to the beach, going to concerts, and going to work. And anxiety about going to the doctor. I had been disbelieved so often that I felt they couldn't help me anymore.

By my mid-30s I had presented to emergency a number of times. I would need morphine and Endone to get me out of the major flare-ups. Still, no-one could tell me what was wrong.

Finally, I had a bit of a breakdown and went to my boss in tears. I told her everything that was happening, and she knew I didn't have much family around, so she kindly gave me the name of her GP, who was an absolute game changer.

I told this amazing GP my story, and we both cried together. She hugged me, then told me she thought I had endometriosis and started organising the tests.

I did a transvaginal ultrasound where they couldn't even see my ovaries because everything was stuck together. My bladder, my uterus and my bowel were all stuck together and were pushing down my ovaries so that they wouldn't even come up on a scan.

The first year after my third laparoscopy was the best year. I was relatively pain free outside of my periods, and I was starting my fertility journey. As we know, endo and adeno severely affect your fertility. I am no exception. In total, we have gone through IVF four times. In seven years I have had eight laparoscopies, four egg-retrieval surgeries and four egg transfers.

Two weeks ago, my partner and I have decided to cease our IVF journey. My endo is out of control still and I haven't been able to manage it for many years. Unfortunately, my body can't take any more of the pain, so I am seeing my specialist and will be pushing to get on the list for a hysterectomy.

It's at this point that I reflected back on my gut instinct all those years ago, which had repeatedly been telling me to freeze my eggs, but doctors wouldn't listen. Had they listened to me all through my twenties, I might have been able to save some better-quality eggs and might have been able to have children today.

Associate Professor Magdalena Simonis AM on symptoms and testing

Associate Professor Magdalena Simonis AM is a GP, government health adviser, board director, primary care researcher with the University of Melbourne, a leading women+'s health expert and gender advocate.

Her interest in endometriosis and persistent pelvic pain began because of the:

> ...recurring presentation of women with misdiagnosed or undiagnosed pelvic pain and heavy menstrual bleeding, stories that were mixed with a variety of vague symptoms and sometimes more obvious menstrual-related problems. Early in my career, we had very little education or training around women's health issues. So, as a graduate...I was uncertain whether to do obstetrics, emergency medicine or general practice.
>
> I did a diploma in obstetrics and gynaecology, and there was so little education about endometriosis and very little about pelvic pain. However, when you go out into the community as a GP, so many women say, 'I have terrible pain with my periods, or I have pain in between my periods. I have pain with sex.' And these were things recurring and reappearing. There was no clear map for GPs who would see many of these young women and older women to ascertain the source of the problems.
>
> When I see these women, who may have heard of endometriosis but don't really understand what it is, I will do a pelvic examination, if they let me. I'll do the swabs, I'll do a physical examination, and I'll take a full history, whether it's a sexual history, health history, menstrual history or a family history if they know of anyone in their family who's had any similar issues.
>
> I also arrange a pelvic ultrasound. I think a pelvic ultrasound is just a really important baseline to determine if there are other issues. They could have fibroids, a bicornuate uterus, an ovarian cyst or other issues. So, it is a baseline investigation.

In outlining what she considers 'normal', she says:

> ... bleeding will go anywhere from one day to five days. That's the common range of a menstrual flow. GPs expect some discomfort with your period that you can manage with a bit of Nurofen or Panadol and a hot water bottle. You can still get on with your day... When you're a young teenager, and you start menstruating, you might have heavier, longer periods than you do when you're 25.

Symptoms are abnormal if you have:

> ... pain that goes beyond day one into day two, day three or four of your menstrual cycle, then that's no longer primary period pain. That is protracted dysmenorrhoea, and even in between periods, it interferes with your ability to do things. Beyond five days, if you're still changing pads frequently, that's a heavy period. Anything beyond eight is abnormal; that is called heavy menstrual bleeding and affects about one in four women. If you do have heavy menstrual bleeding, you have a one in two chance of having endometriosis or some other condition that needs to be addressed.
>
> Suppose your periods go for up to eight days, and you're changing pads or tampons every couple of hours, passing clots that are the size of 50-cent pieces, saturating your sheets and your bedclothes at night with some bleeding, and, you know. In that case, it goes through a pad, goes through two pads—please don't use tampons at night—you've got to get up and change pads, then that's way too heavy. If you can't predict the day ahead and you have to use maybe more than five or six pads in a day, that's heavy menstrual bleeding.
>
> HMB can lead to anaemia, low iron, tiredness and feeling really washed out. That fatigue over a long period of time, if it is not treated, can make you feel quite sad, depressed and lethargic, and you're not able to participate in things fully. Too many young women walk around saying, 'I feel so tired. No matter how much I sleep, I still feel tired in the mornings.' If you're waking up feeling really tired and have periods that go for more than five to seven or eight days, then think about your iron stores.

Dr Tarana Lucky on tests at the gyno

We met Dr Tarana in Chapter 4. Here she gets into more detail on how she approaches the diagnostic process.

> *I want to learn the day-to-day, quality-of-life impacts when you experience period pain and sometimes feel pain that is not easy to define. It might be in the lower abdominal areas, cramps or back pain—endometriosis can give you a range of symptoms.*

Dr Lucky uses three main components for assessment: the first is the patient history and questionnaire responses, and the second she calls the 'bedside evaluation', even if they are in her consulting room.

> *I often start by looking at the patient. Is there overall distress and anxiety from chronic suffering and their experience with pain? Often, my patients cry and are so vulnerable when I talk to them because it's just listening to them that makes them very emotional. Moreover, I hear from 90 per cent of my patients that listening is so important for them.*

Next, she starts the hands-on examination by being 'patient with the patient', and taking a stepped approach.

> *I am reassuring them, first of all, creating a safe space for that examination because I find those living with endometriosis and pelvic pain often would have some trauma history as well. I always start in the least invasive way, such as just feeling their tummy with an abdominal examination and slowly then approaching, with consent and privacy, through to the internal examination.*

When Dr Lucky does the internal examination, there are different components.

> *Starting with the internal vaginal examination, which focuses on feeling or assessing deep disease or deep nodules. I assess the muscle tone, and we call it a myofascial assessment; this is your muscles, and the fascia is connective tissue. Often, depending on the patient's symptoms and history, I may also need to do a transrectal*

60 The Australian Guide to Living Well with Endometriosis

examination. I am always mindful that what I do should not create another traumatic experience for the patient, letting them know 'you can tell me to stop any time', taking it ever so slowly depending on the patient's circumstances.

Sometimes, I do a bit of desensitising and priming movement before I do the internal. Just a bit of like massage or like, know, I make it fun for my patients to make sure they know that it's a safe space, there is nothing to worry about, it is not going to be painful. If it is painful, we will not proceed. The examinations don't all need to be on the one day; we make another appointment and get to know each other.

Asked about the impact of the news.com.au About Bloody Time campaign, which resulted in patients being able to access a longer gynaecologist specialist consultation and have it covered by Medicare, she said:

I cannot stress enough how much this is a game changer. My appointments are always 45 minutes, if not one hour, and sometimes it can overwhelm my patients. We can pick up where we left off in our next review.

Dr Lucky says she supports the multidisciplinary, patient-centred approach.

I'll talk about building their team and suggest they can benefit from pelvic floor physiotherapy, a pain psychologist or a pain specialist, a dietitian. It may be that they choose one at a time, depending on their most impactful symptom and what's their main goal in the short-term and long-term.

She reiterates that the patient should not feel overwhelmed.

Perhaps they start with one team member beside me, to follow through over the next few months. A graded approach is more useful for chronic pain patients. I am also aware of the cost. I think exploring value build options for patients is always important, as is knowing what options are in the public system. Not surprisingly, many of

What to expect from examinations and tests   **61**

these patients are young, starting their careers. Not everyone has private health insurance.

Patients should also be directed to evidence-based websites with resources to help them manage symptoms, like EndoZone. 'Our goal is for patients to manage symptoms themselves, with our guidance', she says.

Ultrasound and MRI are other diagnostic tools, and she notes that laparoscopy used to be the gold standard for diagnosis:

We are no longer taking that invasive approach for diagnosis. If anyone is having a suspected endometriosis, of course, history and examination are the first line. However, also a good imaging evaluation is so important, [as long as it is] undertaken by a quality provider and gynaecologists certified in pelvic ultrasound. Subsidies are available through Medicare and rebates that, unfortunately, some doctors and gynaecologists don't use and should; the patient doesn't need to be out of pocket.

As we talked about before, make sure you have the correct Item number to claim MRI and Ultrasound from Medicare.

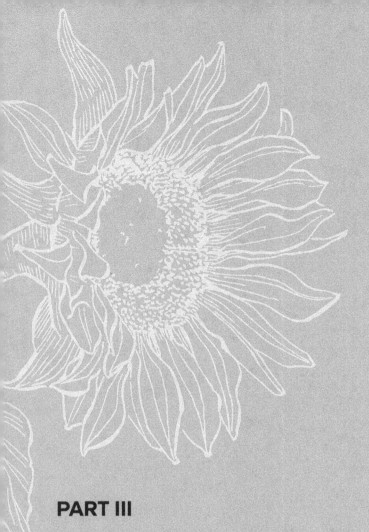

PART III
Treat
Considering your options

CHAPTER 6

What are my treatment options?

There is no cure for endometriosis, but there are several options to help manage the symptoms of pain and heavy menstrual bleeding, and to improve fertility.

Not all therapies work for everyone; individual responses can vary, and you may benefit from combining treatments. We have discussed multidisciplinary care, an integrated approach that involves a team of health practitioners from various medical, allied and integrative health fields working collaboratively to provide comprehensive care for patients.

We will explore the what, why and wherefores of pain medication, hormone treatments and complementary and alternative medicines, which research and evidence suggest can assist you to live well with endometriosis.

Over-the-counter medications

Menstrual, cyclical and other pain can be relieved with over-the-counter medicines. Sometimes, doctors may prescribe stronger pain relief, but these can have side effects, like headaches, stomach and digestive system upsets, asthma, blood pressure, circulation and bleeding problems. It's important to remember that while these medications can help manage pain, they don't treat the underlying endometriosis. There are a number of different medications that may be prescribed for pain, including the following options.

Analgesics

Paracetamol (Acetaminophen), which you may also know as Dymadon, Lemsip, Panadol, Panamax and Tylenol relieves pain and fever but is not anti-inflammatory. Never take more than the recommended dose.

Some also include codeine, such as Panadeine Forte and Panamax Co, while others contain codeine and doxylamine, such as Mersyndol and Mersyndol Forte Panalgesic.

Non-steroidal anti-inflammatories

In Australia, you can obtain these anti-inflammatories with a doctor's prescription or buy lower-dose forms over the counter in a pharmacy. They include aspirin, naproxen, ibuprofen, diclofenac and COX-2 inhibitors (such as celecoxib and meloxicam). They can cause gastro intestinal disturbances and are not recommended if you have asthma.

Palmitoylethanolamide (PEA)

This is a naturally occurring fatty acid amide. It has been found to help with neuropathic and inflammatory pain and the treatment of chronic pain. No major side effects have been attributed to PEA in any study; however, the Therapeutic Goods Administration (TGA) recommends it not be used for more than 21 consecutive days.

Prescription medications

There are several other prescription medical treatments in the doctor's toolkit. These help manage short-term or acute pain by changing the way the nerves communicate pain to the brain, as we talked about on page 18.

Be prepared

You will have heard about opioids and how addictive they can be. They can also have serious side effects; you need to use them just as the doctor or pharmacist tells you to.

Be aware

Opioids include tramadol, buprenorphine, codeine, fentanyl, hydromorphone, methadone, morphine, tapentadol and oxycodone, the latter being commonly prescribed for endometriosis.

Oxycodone

Common brands include Endone, OxyContin and OxyNorm. It comes in different dosages and forms, including tablets, capsules, suppositories and liquid. It can cause breathing problems and constipation, headaches or dizziness, fatigue or drowsiness, loss of appetite, nausea and vomiting.

It *does not* have a place in treating long-term, chronic pain. You may become dependent on this medicine even if you take it exactly as prescribed by your doctor. Your doctor will monitor how you use oxycodone to reduce your risk of harm, including through misuse, abuse and addiction.

Neuromodulators

These can include dopamine, serotonin and endocannabinoids, which communicate between the brain and the body. Be aware they can cause drowsiness and dizziness. However, according to the RANZCOG (gynaecologists) guideline, 'there are no studies evaluating the effectiveness of anti-neuropathic medications for endometriosis-related pain'.

Hormonal treatments

While there is no cure for endo, hormone-based treatments that regulate estrogen are effective for managing the pain and other symptoms experienced with endometriosis. While they can be used as contraceptive birth control, they are also medications that can effectively manage endometriosis symptoms and improve the quality of life for most girls and women+. These therapies aim to help by:

- slowing down or suppressing the growth of endometriosis
- stopping any bleeding (although sometimes there is spotting)
- decreasing inflammation.

The choice of treatment should be made in consultation with your health practitioner, considering your personal circumstances and preferences.

Medications containing a combination of estrogen and progestin, such as combined oral contraceptives, can control periods and suppress endometriosis activity. Progestin-only treatments, including pills, injections, implants and intrauterine devices, prevent endometrial growth and reduce pain.

However, both these types of hormone treatments often have side effects that can lead to women+ stopping the treatment, such as pain persistence, weight gain, spotting and (in very rare cases) blood clots.

Why are they prescribing the pill?

When you finally accept that your pain isn't normal, that it is impacting your life and you find a medical practitioner who listens to you and suggests treatment, it is usually the common pill.

This can be confronting, especially for young girls and women+ from culturally diverse and religiously conservative backgrounds. The concerns include the stigma and presumption of sexual activity and confusion about why a contraceptive pill is being prescribed. You're there for pain and other symptoms, not to prevent pregnancy.

Hormonal treatments aim to decrease the natural ovarian production of estrogens to stop 'feeding' the endometriosis lesions. They suppress the normal menstrual cycle, slow or stop endometriosis growth and may reduce endometriosis-related pain.

Professor Danielle Mazza AO, who we met in Chapter 4, notes that while the pill is a common treatment option for women+, there needs to be a conversation around why the pill is being prescribed and how it can (and can't help) symptoms:

> *Many women often say the GP just told them to take the pill and then sent them home. That perhaps reflects that more of a conversation needs to occur in consultations about why the pill is*

recommended, what endometriosis is, what physiology is and how hormonal medication, which happens to be contraception, actually can assist in changing this trajectory of endometriosis.

We need to explain better that this is a medicine that suppresses estrogen, why it is important and what lesions are. It is challenging, and I think, particularly for a person to be given a contraceptive in non-English speaking background settings and conservative religious settings is even more challenging. The pill is linked only to contraception in some communities; however, it contains hormones that can improve the symptoms by suppressing the tissue and relieving the woman of many things [symptoms] she's presenting with. The fact that it's contraception may be of use to the woman or not relevant to her. It is up to the individual.

Hormone treatment options

Here's a summary of the different types of hormone treatment options your doctor may recommend, including advice from the guide the doctors use from the Australian TGA and the European Society of Human Reproduction and Embryology (ESHRE).

Combined oral contraceptive pill

The oral contraceptive pill (OCP) helps control hormones, reduces endometrial tissue growth and makes periods lighter and less painful. They are often used as a first-line treatment. You'll be directed to take one tablet daily in number order at about the same time each day, without any breaks. It is generally well tolerated, can be stopped quickly and has the additional effect of preventing pregnancy. The OCP can increase the risk of high blood pressure, and, according to the TGA, blood clots. Blood clots are very rare and reported as two cases in every 10000 women+ per year. ESHRE recommends prescribing women+ a combined hormonal contraceptive to reduce endometriosis-associated period, sex and non-menstrual-related pain for continuous use. Your specialist may advise you to skip the sugar pills, which is safe to do and can stop your period completely, relieving symptoms.

Progesterone-like hormones

These hormones come in various forms, including tablets; long-acting injections (depo injections); implants; and intrauterine devices (IUDs) like the Mirena, a small, T-shaped device placed in the uterus, which releases a hormone similar to progesterone.

This helps reduce the activity and pain of endometriosis over time. Long-acting reversible contraception (LARC) can stop menstruation and is generally well tolerated; it does not require further interventions, such as daily dosing or monthly administration, with the option of removal at any time. The TGA has extended its lifespan to eight years.

Oral progestins

Visanne (dienogest) is an oral progestin used for treating endometriosis. While it shares some characteristics with other progestins, there are important distinctions: Visanne is not a contraceptive and should not be used for birth control. If contraception is required while taking Visanne, discuss this with your doctor — a non-hormonal method such as condoms or other barrier methods should be used.

It is generally well-tolerated, but side effects can occur. Visanne may cause changes in menstrual bleeding, including irregular bleeding or spotting. Common side effects include headache, breast discomfort, acne, nausea and weight gain. Mood changes and decreased libido can also occur.

Visanne (dienogest) has officially been added to the Pharmaceutical Benefits Scheme (PBS) in Australia for the treatment of endometriosis, effective December 1, 2024. This is a significant milestone, marking the first new medication for endometriosis to be included in the PBS in three decades.

GnRH agonists

GnRH agonists are injections and nasal sprays that can stop the release of reproductive hormones, which might lead to a menopause-like state that many women+ find uncomfortable. It can cause hot flushes, night sweats and increases risks associated with decreased bone density. These medications are usually not used alone for more than a few months due to potential long-term side effects. They block ovulation and periods, and are very effective in reducing pain related to endometriosis. Taking this treatment stops endometriosis growth in most cases. The PBS subsidises only six months of treatment and, after this, the medication becomes expensive. The use of additional hormone therapy is common, adding to the burden of treatment.

GnRH antagonists

GnRH antagonist Ryeqo is the new player on the court. It is the first endometriosis treatment approved by the TGA in Australia for 13 years, and the first oral GnRH antagonist combination therapy in Australia. It comes in a tablet or a medicine bottle, unlike the very obvious 'pill pack', so there is less stigma for those from culturally and religiously conservative families. It contains lower doses of estrogen and progestogen than those used in combined hormonal contraceptives, and is provided in combination with relugolix, a molecule that reduces estrogen and other hormones in the body.

Ryeqo was recommended for the PBS subsidy for endometriosis treatment in 2024, which will significantly reduce the cost, making it accessible and affordable. At the time of writing, it can be used for up to two years, then continued at the prescriber's discretion. It has been used to treat fibroids for several years.

Ryeqo is a contraceptive, and you need to stop using any other hormonal contraception when you start taking it, using a barrier method in the first month while it settles in. Ovulation returns, along with menstrual bleeding, the month you stop taking it, which is great if you're trying to fall pregnant naturally or going through assisted reproductive technology (ART) and IVF. Like other hormone suppression, bone mineral density needs to be monitored, and a baseline DEXA (bone density) assessment is recommended at the start of treatment and then annually.

The clinical trials showed very similar incidences of hot flushes in those taking the medicine and the inactive placebo.

Be aware

Always seek medical advice before taking medications and report any side effects to your treating doctor immediately.

Be prepared

As the GPs have explained, you need to stick with these treatments for a few months unless there are serious effects.

Medicinal cannabis

Cannabis, AKA marijuana, joint, weed, reefer, doobie, good giggles, wisdom weed, pot, 710 is ingested in a session, 420, vape, hot box to make users toasted, baked, mashed, fried, stoned, high and wasted.

It grows between a policy wasteland and a medical minefield, and carries a stigma that users are stoners and potheads. Using cannabis in any form remains illegal in Australia unless prescribed by a healthcare or medical practitioner.

The Federal Department of Health and Aged Care tells us: 'Cultivation, manufacture, importation and exportation of medicinal cannabis is tightly controlled by the Office of Drug Control, the TGA and local state and territories.' Better Health Channel in Victoria describes it as 'the most commonly used illegal drug'.

So what's the buzz?

It has been known for millennia that cannabis has healing properties and, in 2016, Australia legalised growing cannabis for medicinal and scientific purposes. In the pain section on page 17, we discussed the endocannabinoid system (ECS)—'missing in action' in women+ with endometriosis—involved in influencing the nervous system and its functions, including regulating pain, inflammation and immune function.

Many studies suggest that the cannabis compounds cannabidiol (CBD) and tetrahydrocannabinol (THC), psychoactive compounds that influence the ECS by altering how the nervous system functions, may help manage symptoms of endometriosis, as well as relieve associated gastrointestinal issues and mood disorders.

A study published in *Gynecologic Endocrinology and Reproductive Medicine* (2024) found that people with endometriosis using cannabis reported a 90 per cent improvement in menstrual pain, and many participants were able to reduce their pain medication intake.

The impact can vary depending on the method of ingestion. Inhaled forms of cannabis were found to work better for pain relief, while oral forms were superior for mood and gastrointestinal symptoms.

Australia has seen a significant increase in the number of prescriptions for medicinal cannabis. By the end of 2022, the TGA reported it had approved over 300 000 prescriptions for medicinal cannabis since it was legalised for medical use in 2016.

72   The Australian Guide to Living Well with Endometriosis

At the time of writing, there are *no* TGA-approved cannabis products for endometriosis and pelvic pain, which means the ones on the market have not been tested for 'safety, quality or effectiveness'. So please keep yourself up to date on developments in this space and learn more through the medicinal cannabis hub online (see the resources section).

Why some women+ choose to use medical cannabis: Rachel's story

Rachel Payne MLC is an endo warrior. Since 2022, she has represented the Legalise Cannabis Victoria party and the South Eastern Melbourne region in the Victorian Parliament. Rachel is well-qualified, with postgraduate qualifications in public policy and an undergraduate degree in sociology and politics. Rachel is one of the loudest voices advocating for change in laws, workplace policies, prescribing, pricing and product quality around cannabis. She says:

So many of the conversations that I've had, particularly with people who use cannabis, have been women much like myself, who have used cannabis for pain relief. And when we do talk about some of the symptoms that you experience, whether it be the physical or some of the ongoing effects of managing pain around endometriosis, those that I have spoken to who have discovered cannabis as a suitable alternative to other medications they have been prescribed have found it rather life changing.

Rachel shares that she 'struggled with pain management with my periods from quite a young age, and it became quite prevalent when I started experiencing more stresses in my life as well'.

For me, and I'm sure this is the experience of most people who are diagnosed with endometriosis, you go through a process of either not feeling heard or being misrepresented when it comes to healthcare. And everyone whom I speak to who has been on that journey, particularly those who now use medicinal cannabis and use it effectively, has found that when you do present to a doctor. You want to have that conversation, and there is a requirement that you have tried every other form of pain medication and relief.

Those who start to use medicinal cannabis find that not only does it provide pain relief but it also has that ongoing lasting impact of anti-inflammatory properties. It can help with symptoms of depression. It can help with symptoms of inflammation and swelling. It can also help with things that encourage mood and provide that relaxation effect.

She is told by many women+ that 'traditional medication that's prescribed starts to lack effectiveness and impact, which means that you start to increase your dose, which can be quite harmful', and says she has:

... spoken to people who have become dependent on those opioids, but they can also have more ongoing effects around mood, around the impacts it can have on your body, on your other organs. Cannabis, on the other hand, has a very low harm profile, yet we don't see that as something that is often prescribed or something that is pointed to. The majority of people I speak to have to discover that for themselves.

She explains the effectiveness of cannabis:

We know that not only is it CBD, which is sort of more of an anti-inflammatory and non-psychoactive component of cannabis, but THC, which is psychoactive but also has an enormous impact when it comes to pain management. Terpene profiles help appetite if someone is taking medication that is causing them to have nausea.

As an elected lawmaker experienced in public policy, she notes that:

As a cannabis community, we are wide and varied, but when it comes to the discussion around cannabis, it's not only the law reform that needs to happen in that space but also the stigma that is attached to those who use cannabis in a medicinal sense. We do find that it is really important to have those conversations that break down those barriers around why people do access cannabis.

Discussing roadside drug testing, she notes:

Road safety has to be an imperative part of this conversation. I'm very mindful of the fact that the road safety issues that we're experiencing in this country are quite prevalent. However, I would argue that it's not medicinal cannabis patients who are causing issues around road safety. I would say mobile phones would have to be number one when it came to the most distracting thing for a driver on the road. CBD as a plant derivative is the non-psychoactive part.

She is also conscious that there is a presumption about the person found to have cannabis in their system:

… they're treated as though they are someone who had just smoked a bong two hours earlier—Johnny, who knocked off work early and decided to have a bit of fun and then jumped in the car… compared with Rachel, who's a 40-something-year-old woman who took her medication last night because she had severe pain. The next day, I'm clearly not impaired, but on a roadside drug test, I could test positive to having THC in my system.

Rachel has 'come out' as a medicinal cannabis user and an endo warrior, and she shares that her role as a Member of Parliament representing the Legalise Cannabis Victoria party has:

… actually helped me make further connections with a lot of other women who are experiencing [symptoms] similar to what I have. I guess it's made me more available to questions about that as well. And I'm really mindful of the fact that not everyone wants to smoke a joint or use a vaporiser. So, even just those conversations around prescription—you can be prescribed a tincture that you can have two drops of a night-time and what relief that will provide you.

Reflecting on what she wants readers to remember, she says:

I think it's really important for us to be vulnerable, to stand up, to share our experiences because it provides an opportunity for others to connect with that story as well.

Be aware

Medicinal cannabis is generally not covered by the PBS, which means patients must pay out of pocket for these treatments. Private health insurance may provide some coverage, but this is not common and coverage varies by provider.

Policy and regulation are playing 'catch up' as the uptake of medicinal cannabis use increases exponentially. In many countries, including Australia, the regulatory framework for medicinal cannabis is still evolving. This creates challenges in quality control, access and cannabis road safety consistency across different jurisdictions.

Be aware

Cannabis may interact with other medications, potentially altering their effects; however, research on these interactions is still limited.

The long-term health effects of regular medicinal cannabis use are not fully understood, particularly when it comes to cognitive function, lung health (for smoked or vaporised forms) and mental health.

Although the risk of dependence and abuse is lower with medicinal use, there is still a concern about the potential for dependence or abuse, particularly when THC is involved.

Traditional and alternative options

For millennia, our First Nations peoples have used plants to treat ailments and illnesses. Increasingly, complementary and alternative medicines, working in conjunction with Western conventional medical treatment, provide a holistic opportunity for managing endometriosis symptoms.

Medicinal herbs

Herbal medicines with anti-inflammatory properties may help with endometriosis pain, but more research is needed. Some of the common herbs that women+ use include:

- turmeric: a powerful anti-inflammatory, which has been shown to have antioxidant and anti-proliferative effects in endometriosis studies
- chamomile: limited research (one study) has shown it contains a compound that suppresses and kills endometrial cells in a lab setting, but more research is required; also has the antioxidant apigenin, which promotes good digestion and sleep
- dandelion: can stimulate appetite, help digestion and enhance kidney function; contains vitamins A, B, C and D, as well as iron, potassium and zinc; high in fructose, so not suitable for those on the FODMAP diet
- lemon balm: alleviates menstrual cramps, relieves nausea and reduces stress and anxiety
- slippery elm: soothes inflammatory bowel conditions, heartburn, sore throats and urinary tract infections.

Chinese herbal medicine

Numerous studies indicate traditional Chinese herbal formulas may decrease lesion size, alleviate pelvic pain and reduce postoperative recurrence in endometriosis patients. Some herbs you may hear discussed by your herbalist may include:

- dong quai: relieves symptoms of premenstrual syndrome, menopause and period cramps by improving blood circulation
- ginger: has antioxidant properties and can reduce nausea as well as relieve inflammatory conditions
- gingko biloba: contains high levels of antioxidants, is anti-inflammatory and helps headaches and migraines
- ginseng: may relieve inflammation and reduce stress
- thunder god vine: has triptolide, a compound with anti-inflammatory properties.

Indian Ayurvedic herbal therapies

Ancient Indian physician Charaka described Ayurveda as 'the knowledge of happy and unhappy, a good and bad life, and that which contributes to those four aspects'. These relate to health in Ayurveda, through:

- doshas, which include Vata (force of movement, activity and sensation), Pitta (source of transformative processes) and Kapha (the body's strength and stability) are also called 'tridoshas'
- dhatus, tissues that make up the body's physical form
- agni, the body's digestive fire
- malas, the body's waste (pee, poo and sweat), which can build up and cause disease.

According to *A conceptual view of endometriosis through an Ayurveda perspective*:

> *Overgrowth of cells is a Kapha imbalance. Since the location of the uterus and involvement of hormones as well as blood, it also indicates a Pitta imbalance. Since menstrual cycle involves movement it is also a Vata disorder. Imbalance of all three Doshas leads to endometriosis, more or less which indicates vitiation or lack of balance in Tridoshas.*

Some herbs that you may hear discussed include:

- boswellia: an anti-inflammatory that helps with inflammatory bowel disease, arthritis and may reduce pelvic pain symptoms
- ashwagandha: may balance hormones, reduce inflammation and support the immune system
- shatavari: may regulate hormone levels, improve fertility and reduce menstrual pain
- curcumin: the active compound in turmeric; has shown anti-inflammatory, antioxidant and anti-proliferative effects in endometriosis studies.

Be aware

While these natural therapies show promise, more research is needed to confirm their effectiveness. It's important to consult with a doctor before starting any new treatments or making significant dietary changes. A combination of natural therapies along with conventional medical treatment may provide the best approach for managing endometriosis symptoms.

As always, be mindful of finding a competent practitioner and consider the quality and safety of whatever you take. Check out the peak bodies for further information, such as Complementary Medicines Australia, which is the peak body for vitamins and minerals, herbal remedies and traditional medicines like Ayurveda and Chinese medicine, and Chinese Medicine Industry Council of Australia Ltd (CMIC) is the peak body representing the importers and suppliers of Chinese Herbal Medicines.

Be prepared

Medicines approved for supply in Australia display an Australian Register of Therapeutic Goods (ARTG) number starting with 'AUST' and followed by an 'R' or L(A). Those with AUST L(A) are assessed for efficacy, while those with AUST L are not.

Better Health Channel warns that Ayurvedic medicines that are not registered with the TGA should be avoided, and there have been cases of serious side effects. To be safe, buy Australian-made complementary medicines which are subject to TGA safety and quality regulations.

CHAPTER 7

Considering surgery

Surgery can be a common outcome for women+ with endometriosis, and may be part of an ongoing treatment plan to manage the pain caused by lesions and adhesions. Surgery may be suggested by your gynaecologist for:

- severe pain: if you experience chronic or debilitating pelvic pain that medication cannot alleviate
- diagnosis confirmation: a laparoscopy (a minimally invasive procedure) can confirm the presence of endometriosis and allow for treatment at the same time
- endometriosis impacting organs: If endometriosis affects surrounding organs like the bowel or bladder, more specialised surgical teams may be involved, including urologists and colorectal surgeons.

The most common surgical approach is laparoscopy, where small incisions are made to remove endometrial tissue. In some cases, a laparotomy (a larger incision) may be necessary for more extensive disease.

Laparoscopic surgery

RANZCOG considers surgery the 'gold standard' for definitive diagnosis of endometriosis, especially if other hormonal treatments are ineffective or inappropriate, and where ultrasound scans seem normal but endometriosis is still suspected.

In Australia, endometriosis is usually removed surgically by cutting (excision) or treated by destroying the cells using diathermy (ablation).

Dr Tarana Lucky explains her approach to laparoscopic procedures:

In surgical excision, it should be once and all as much as possible. If you have a partial excision, that's no good because there is a higher chance of recurrence, adhesion and scarring. There are three situations when I would do surgery for those patients. One, they have tried different types of hormones, have failed, and [their symptoms] are still having a significant impact on... their quality of life... Number two, some patients feel like they need the answer, although I tell them that we do not do the surgery for diagnosis. However, they're suffering, despite long-term hormone therapy, and they seek the validation that they have endometriosis. I tell them it will not be for diagnosis, and the third group is sometimes for patients having trouble with fertility and conception. For every patient, the day before surgery, I would go through their history, imaging, MRI, reflect on their main goal based on a discussion I had with the patient.

She uses the belly button as the entry point to:

... have a thorough look everywhere where those cheeky lesions are, and that involves the diaphragm, looking under the liver, because the upper abdomen is rare but a place where endometriosis can deposit. After the mapping, I would decide what areas to approach for excision and then find a fine balance between the ovaries and normal organs versus the lesions. As much as possible, excision with a healthy margin is the best way to remove the disease.

Once she has mapped the area through the belly button hole with a camera, she already knows what stage of endometriosis she's dealing with (one to four).

If I have the robotic platform available, I can see in 3D, and the lesions are clear, which means a higher identification rate, and I decide how many ports I need. The port placement is slightly different for robotic cases [compared with] routine laparoscopy, but the number varies between three to five ports. But they're all very small. They're less than 1 centimetre, most of the time between 5 to 8 millimetres.

Using robotics, in my experience, for major surgeries like complex stage 4 endo, [lets] my patients go home the same day. They have shorter recoveries, less of a pain score and less blood loss compared with a traditional approach. This is based on my own observations; there isn't enough data.

One reason for this is that with the robotic approach, you can use less intraperitoneal pressure [the cavity space inside the abdomen and pelvis that is surrounded by a layer of tissue]. I need less air because the vision is clear without it.

You have much more opportunity for wrist-like manipulation. In laparoscopy, for example, you could move it [the robotics] 360 degrees ... whenever there is a tricky angle to find that lesion.

Second, the movement we do in the port often [uses] a traditional stretch stick, which puts a lot of pressure on the patient's skin. With the robot arm, they have this pivot end that ... adjusts that angle. Thirdly, the vision is so meticulous and 3D that the tissue injury is less in robotics, the bleeding is less, and subsequently, that creates a less painful experience in the recovery.

For patients who want to have the best chance at pregnancy, she is mindful of whether ovarian cysts need full excision or draining:

It all depends on the patient's fertility journey. After the excision, ensuring good haemostasis [stopping the bleeding] is a part of adhesion control for the future. Some anti-adhesion barriers are available, and I use the products with stronger data.

She explains that they come in different forms, like a spray gel or a light filmy product, and can be made of different substances, like cellulose or similar. They stay there, sealing the area.

They prevent the bowel or other organs from getting stuck onto the lesions where I have done the excision, because, naturally, our body heals by fibrosis [scarring], but we are trying to keep that area separate from the other organs.

She explained that the robotic platform gives her 'three arms', which help her 'get into that back little corner behind the uterus or in that awkward corner behind the bowel, and I can have access to three arms that I can use simultaneously'.

However, surgery is not a cure: relapse of symptoms occurs in 40 to 45 per cent of women+, while around 30 per cent of women+ are readmitted for surgery within five years.

Not all experts agree about surgery...

Surgery is a necessary diagnostic and treatment pathway for lesions and adhesions that are causing excruciating pain, the medical term used to describe stage 4 endometriosis. It is also required when endometrial implants impact other organs, including the bladder, bowel, rectum and ovaries. Sometimes ovarian cysts burst and require surgical intervention or fallopian tubes are abnormal due to endometriosis or damage from previous surgeries.

The Faculty of Pain Medicine of the Australian and New Zealand College of Anaesthetists, supported by Private Healthcare Australia, suggests surgery is a 'waste of money' that may worsen outcomes for some women+, through complications such as infections, damage to organs like the bowel and bladder, and blood vessel damage. It argues that 'Endometriosis is found in only 40 to 60 per cent of laparoscopies in people who have persistent pelvic pain ... but lesions are also found in up to 45 per cent of pain-free women', and that 50 per cent of women+ who have laparoscopic surgery to find the source of their disease are found to have no lesions. According to Professor Sonia Grover, the patients 'had endured an invasive surgery that had its own risks and invalidated their pain even further'.

We have discussed a patient-centred approach and rights, including the right to accurate, relevant information to make informed healthcare and treatment decisions. We will expand on this in the next part of the book. If you are not sure about the benefits of surgery or have concerns about the costs and risks, discuss this with your gynaecologist. You can always ask for a second opinion.

Hysterectomy

Studies indicate that only about 25 per cent of women+ experience significant pain relief after a hysterectomy. For the remaining 75 per cent, pain may persist or worsen, especially if the ovaries are retained, as endometriosis can still occur outside the uterus.

Hysterectomy rates for endometriosis have been decreasing in Australia, but it remains a procedure that some women+ undergo, especially when other treatments have failed for adenomyosis.

According to the Royal Women's Hospital in Melbourne, hysterectomy and endometriosis removal achieve a long-term cure in over 90 per cent of women+ and, as a result, reduce or eliminate the need to use medications long-term. They stop periods and end fertility. However, it does not cure endometriosis, as the condition can reoccur even after the removal of the uterus, especially if endometrial tissue remains elsewhere in the body.

There are two types of hysterectomy:

1. total hysterectomy: removal of the uterus and cervix
2. sub-total hysterectomy: removal of the uterus only, leaving the cervix in place.

There are three ways in which a hysterectomy can be performed:

1. Abdominal hysterectomy: An operation is performed through the abdomen. This will require an incision (cut) to be made in the lower part of your abdomen to allow the gynaecologist to operate.
2. Vaginal hysterectomy: is the removal of the uterus through the vagina, with no need for any incisions through the abdomen.
3. Laparoscopic hysterectomy: This hysterectomy is performed under the guidance of a special camera that passes through a keyhole in the abdomen, while other instruments pass through separate keyholes.

Be prepared

At the time of hysterectomy, one or both of the ovaries may be removed. It is also common for one or both of the fallopian tubes to be removed. The type of hysterectomy and whether the ovaries or fallopian tubes are removed will depend on your personal circumstances. Your gynaecologist will discuss it with you before your operation.

Be aware

A hysterectomy means you will not be able to carry a baby, and this can lead to a sense of loss and grief for unfulfilled hopes of motherhood. It may also not cure pain associated with endometriosis, where tissue similar to the lining of the uterus grows elsewhere, particularly in the pelvic cavity.

The decision to have a hysterectomy: Anna's story

Anna Thomas is a teacher, and despite it being a 'feminised profession', the reality of managing heavy menstrual bleeding and pain in a primary school classroom is challenging for this endo warrior.

I am 35 and have severe endometriosis. I was diagnosed at age 22, although I have been dealing with pain since age 12. I was living in Tasmania, and my first laparoscopic surgery at 23 didn't go well. I was sent to Melbourne, and the surgeon said I had much more endometriosis than he would expect in a person my age. He removed as much of the endo as possible, working alongside a colorectal surgeon who removed a section of my bowel.

The surgery was successful, and we were given a 10 per cent chance of naturally falling pregnant. My husband and I were beyond blessed, and we introduced our baby boy to the world in 2014. It was a miracle and something we never realistically thought would happen for us.

Unfortunately, my endometriosis came back with a vengeance, and I had to try a variety of medications. I was on a hormonal roller-coaster.

After a few years of treatment, I was able to try for a second child, and I became pregnant with our darling baby. We miscarried at 12 weeks in 2017, but he is forever part of our family. We love him dearly and never a day goes by that we don't think of him.

We were given one last window of hope — a 2 per cent chance of falling pregnant again, and we welcomed our third child in 2018 after a very rocky pregnancy and delivery. Another miracle!

Being a teacher and living with endometriosis is a daily struggle. Needing to take time off work is a constant hit to the bank account, and not just physically tough but mentally, too. Between the severe bleeding, aches, pains, throbbing, cramping, migraines, bloating, brain fog and many more symptoms, it's a hell of suffering and stress to my body.

In early 2024, my endometriosis symptoms seemed to be increasing in severity, and it was time for another internal scan and check-up with my new specialist. It showed I needed to have a hysterectomy, something I have been trying to avoid for the past five years. The pill I have been on since age 22 had created a blood 'bubble' in my uterus, meaning that I couldn't even do a ten-minute walk without bleeding. Bike riding or any strenuous activity would mean an instant bleed, and sometimes, I didn't even get a chance to get to a bathroom.

I had major surgery consisting of a total robotic hysterectomy, resection of endometriosis of my ovaries and bowel, cystoscopy, and much more. I needed a full eight weeks of recovery — two steps forward, one step backwards.

Having endometriosis is not just a strain on me but also on my husband and children, who are by my side, loving and supporting me. They are the ones who have handed me sanitary items, got me pain medication and a heat pack, and picked me up off the *bathroom floor when I've nearly collapsed from the pain. It affects all those who love and support you, as they are living it with you and going through all that having the disease entails.*

I am now off the majority of my medication, as I felt I needed some time off it to be able to work out the new me. But that comes with its issues, such as severe cramping, as the medication is used to suppress the pain.

All those living with endo—we are fighters, and we need to work together to do all we can to support others with the disease and educate the community.

CHAPTER 8

Fertility and infertility

According to the World Health Organization, one in six couples experience infertility. Many can improve their chances with lifestyle changes or be successfully treated with surgical techniques and ART.

I had IVF for my youngest daughter. I was a Member of Parliament in my 20s with two children, and I was determined to have another baby. Fertility treatment is challenging, and even without endometriosis, I found the hormones and injections gave me awful hot flushes. I was moodier than I had ever felt in my life, before or since, and that was challenging for those around me! I remember apologising for saying something outrageous — 'Sorry, that was the hormones talking' — and my husband said, 'That doesn't make it right. I love you.' I cried uncontrollably for hours, upsetting the kids who were nine and six at the time.

You'll hear from many women+ in their late teens or early twenties who are diagnosed with endometriosis and how horrified their mothers were when the GP or gynaecologist told them to have a baby as soon as possible. That advice can be confusing and sounds flippant and disrespectful to your life plans, which may not include a baby. However, this advice comes from a place of knowledge, concern and empathy.

Females are born with between one and two million eggs, and you don't grow any more. The number of eggs decreases when you ovulate, which triggers periods. You are most fertile during your 20s;

from 30, fertility drops off until menopause. After menopause, it is not possible to get pregnant naturally.

Most women+ have menstrual cycles of 23 to 35 days; after ovulation, your period arrives 12 to 16 days later. This is the best time to get that sperm and egg to have a meet-and-greet and create magic together.

My daughter and her now-husband were given the same advice by the most wonderful, caring gynaecologist when they were in their early 20s. They didn't need IVF in the end, conceiving naturally right at the six-month mark, when IVF was the next option on the agenda. Brianna is now working as a fertility nurse.

Bindi Irwin, who released information about her endometriosis journey in March 2023, made a poignant statement in September 2024 when asked about having another child.

> *... you never know what's happening in someone's life or in a family's world ... everything may seem fine on the outside and on the inside, their own personal journey might've been filled with turmoil and challenges ... many, many people ... can't have another baby, can't have a baby at all. (Kidspot 2024)*

How does endo impact fertility?

Endometriosis impacts fertility in a number of ways. The inflammation that causes pain and bleeding can also reduce egg quality. It may be associated with implantation failure and an increased risk of miscarriage.

It is an uncomfortable truth that age decreases your chances of having a baby, with research indicating that around a third of women+ with endometriosis experience infertility, and an estimated 50 per cent of infertile patients doing IVF and ART are found to have endometriosis.

Difficulty getting pregnant can be an early sign of something. Endometriosis can affect fertility by damaging the ovaries where the eggs are and the fallopian tubes that transport them through anatomic distortions and scarring, which can block fallopian tubes and prevent the eggs from combining with sperm.

Endometriosis lesions, scarring and adhesions in the pelvic area affect the overall fertility environment. Adenomyosis also impacts the uterus, where the embryo needs to implant and stay to grow.

The relationship between endometriosis and infertility is complex, and the mechanisms by which endometriosis affects fertility are not fully understood. However, it is believed that inflammation; altered immune system functioning; changes in the hormonal environment of the reproductive tract; and mechanical factors, such as adhesions, may all play a role.

Many women+ are not even aware they have endometriosis or adenomyosis until they seek medical help because they are not conceiving naturally. Sometimes, if you've been on the pill to avoid getting pregnant, it may have actually masked endometriosis symptoms, and you don't realise it is affecting you until you stop taking contraceptives or seek medical help for infertility.

Coming off your medications

If you have been diagnosed with endo and adeno, you've probably spent years on the pill or using other hormone treatments to manage your endometriosis symptoms. So what happens when that little voice in your head tells you to make a baby? Chances are, coming off the medications (hormones) treating your endo and adeno will cause heavy bleeding and painful sex—neither create the 'vibe' for making a baby. Your pelvic pain may return with a vengeance, along with joint pain, headaches or migraines, acne, hair loss and brain fog.

Generally, your menstrual cycle will return to whatever is 'normal' for you after you stop hormones. It's important to take this into account as there may be a delay between when you stop taking the contraceptive (or have it removed) and when you can conceive. Here are some of the contraceptive types and how long they take to stop working once you stop taking them:

- oral contraceptive pill: about two months
- progestin-only (also known as the mini pill): very quickly, usually within a month
- Ryeqo: generally in a month
- hormone-releasing intrauterine device (IUD; e.g. Mirena): you can get pregnant immediately or sometime in the first year

Fertility and infertility **91**

- contraception implant: within a month
- contraception injection: between eight and 12 months, although this may be longer in some individuals
- vaginal ring: one to three months after removal.

> ### Be prepared
>
> If you are even thinking about pregnancy, going off hormonal treatment and contraceptives, start taking supplements with folate to support the baby's development. To increase your chances of conceiving and improve your baby's health, as well as your own, take DHA, an omega-3 fatty acid, especially if you don't eat fish or are vegetarian.

What to expect from a fertility specialist

The Fertility Society of Australia and New Zealand suggest that, if you are under 35, you should see a GP or fertility specialist if you've been trying to conceive for 12 months. If you're over 35, seek advice after six months of trying.

Being asked about your sex life and lifestyle can be really confronting for you and your partner. You'll be asked things like how often you have sex; which positions you use; how long you've been trying to conceive; which contraceptives (hormone treatments) you've been on, for how long, and about any side effects; whether you have regular periods; if you are up to date with cervical screening (recommended from the age of 25); whether you have had any sexually transmitted infections, and so on.

They will also ask for a maternal family history of endometriosis, miscarriages, infertility and hysterectomy. You'll both also be asked about lifestyle, and be honest: Do you smoke or take drugs, including cannabis and anything else from mushrooms to meth? How much alcohol and caffeine do you consume? Have you been exposed to any chemicals or toxins, especially regularly? What do you weigh? Have you gained or lost weight? Do you exercise, what and how often? Are you stressed?

You'll probably be referred for blood tests for hormones, including follicle-stimulating hormone (FSH), luteinising hormone (LH), and your level of anti-Mullerian hormone (AMH), an indicator of your ovarian reserve. You will have a cervix swab to check for chlamydia and a urine test.

You may be referred for a pelvic ultrasound to check your ovaries, uterus and fallopian tubes and to detect endometriosis. Conditions like fibroids may be detected, as well as signs of blocked or damaged fallopian tubes. If the ultrasound suggests possible blockage, you will be referred for a hysterosalpingo-contrast-ultrasonography (HyCoSy) or an x-ray. You may have a laparoscopy to examine your uterus, fallopian tubes and ovaries.

Fertility treatment options

Treatment options for infertility related to endometriosis include laparoscopic surgery, ovarian stimulation to produce as many eggs as possible and prepare them for release, followed by Intrauterine insemination (IUI), with healthy sperm placed in the uterus around the time of ovulation; Intracytoplasmic sperm injection (ICSI), with sperm injected directly into each egg; and in vitro fertilisation (IVF), when an egg is fertilised by sperm in a test tube or elsewhere outside the body.

Freezing your eggs

If you are concerned about endo and adeno impacting your fertility, have had ovarian reserve tests or have been told chocolate cysts have damaged your ovaries, you can explore egg freezing to help preserve your future fertility. When you're ready to use your eggs, they are thawed and fertilised before being implanted into your uterus.

Donor eggs

Ovarian reserve tests help a doctor estimate the number of eggs a woman+ has. If the number is low, the person may consider using donor eggs to conceive. Egg donation is regulated in Australia by the National Health and Medical Research Council's (NHMRC) Ethical Guidelines and the Code of Practice of the Reproductive Technology Accreditation Committee of the Fertility Society of Australia.

These regulations ensure that the process of egg donation adheres to ethical standards and promotes the welfare of all parties involved, including donors and recipients. The regulations emphasise informed consent, donor anonymity (where applicable), and donors' psychological and physical health. They also address issues related to donor compensation, ensuring it is appropriate and not coercive.

Starting the IVF process

The first step in exploring IVF as an option is to discuss your fertility concerns with your GP. You will need a referral to a fertility specialist — if you don't have a preferred specialist, your doctor can suggest a clinic. You can ask your GP for an 'indefinite' referral so you are eligible for Medicare rebates. As long as you have a valid referral, there is no limit on the number of treatment rounds.

Unless you are accepted into a public health IVF service, you will be paying some costs yourself, depending on the services you use, the cost of your fertility specialist and clinic, and the level of private health insurance cover, if you have it. Each state and territory have their own regulations around funding for ART, including IVF. Some states, such as Queensland, Victoria and New South Wales, will publicly fund ART (and that includes fertility preservation services) for people with complex medical conditions, such as cancer. South Australia, Northern Territory and Tasmania do not provide public IVF services.

Costs

If you are not eligible for or don't have access to IVF in the public health system, typical costs for IVF treatment can be significant. Even with private health insurance, you will likely be out of pocket thousands of dollars per cycle. Please check your eligibility for IVF coverage and ask your health fund for a quote for rebates ahead of booking your IVF treatment. Many IVF providers have their costs on their websites, which may assist you in choosing a provider and planning for the likely costs. There may also be additional fees charged by some clinics for beds and medication costs.

Next steps in the IVF journey

Once you have decided to undergo IVF, there are specific medications and procedures required for a hopefully successful implantation of an embryo.

- Ovarian hyperstimulation: You take fertility medications, such as FSH and LH, to stimulate the ovaries to produce more eggs for collection and fertilisation.
- Egg retrieval: Under general anaesthesia, a fertility doctor uses an ultrasound to guide a long, thin needle through the vaginal wall into the ovarian follicles. A suction device attached to the needle retrieves the eggs from the follicles.
- Insemination and fertilisation: The retrieved eggs are prepared for fertilisation. They are either placed with sperm to allow natural fertilisation or injected directly with sperm through a procedure called intracytoplasmic sperm injection.
- Embryo culture: The fertilised eggs divide and grow over five to seven days, reaching the blastocyst stage (meaning the embryo is a ball of cells). At this point, pre-implantation genetic testing can be performed to ensure the embryo has a normal number of chromosomes.
- Embryo transfer: Once the embryo reaches the blastocyst stage, it can be transferred into the uterus. This can be done either as a fresh transfer (without freezing) or during a frozen embryo transfer cycle. A single embryo is typically transferred, but the number can vary based on several factors, including your personal circumstances, which you will discuss with your fertility specialist.
- Pregnancy begins at implantation when the embryo attaches to the uterine lining.

Professor Luk Rombauts on how endo impacts fertility

Professor Luk Rombauts is the past president of the World Endometriosis Society and presided over the Edinburgh 2023 World Congress on Endometriosis (WCE). I am honoured to be on the organising committee with him for the Sydney WCE. He has been with Monash IVF Group for almost 24 years. He discussed how women+'s fertility is affected by endometriosis and how it's a fine balance between treating endo with hormones and creating the optimal environment for pregnancy.

> *The hormonal treatments are all based on suppressing the menstrual cycle. That will stop the endometrium, the lining inside the uterus, from growing thick. However, given that endometriosis is a very similar tissue, it will also prevent the growth of the endometriotic lesions. The problem with that is that we have a large group of women still very much in their reproductive years who need to treat their endometriosis pain but also want to start a family.*
>
> *Ideally, these molecules wouldn't interfere with the woman's reproductive cycle if these women are trying to start a family. As coming off hormone treatment for endo is unpredictable, we can't be sure when ovulation occurs. You don't know when you're in early pregnancy. We want to ensure the development of the growing foetus isn't at risk.*

When discussing fertility preservation, many women+ are unaware their infertility is related to endometriosis until it is investigated.

> *If you've got extensive endometriosis on your ovaries, it depends on the skills of the surgeon to make sure there's as little damage as possible because that's where your egg reserve resides... Unfortunately, any surgery to your ovary will diminish that ovarian reserve. So, if you've got repetitive surgery, in particular, you will find that your egg reserve will decline quite dramatically.*

Professor Rombauts echoes the advice that many women+ hear from doctors urging them to have children sooner rather than later.

> *Generally, as fertility specialists, we say to all women, 'If you're in a position to start a family, start it right now. Don't delay: your eggs decline in number but also in quality.'*
>
> *I don't want to scare patients too much, but there certainly have been cases where an ovary on one side goes into menopause. So, it is*

vital that you ask your surgeon, 'What would the potential impact be on my egg reserve? Do you think that I'm at the stage where perhaps I should consider preserving my fertility?'

For many with endometriosis, based on my review of the literature and the evidence, there is a diminishing likelihood of falling pregnant naturally … But once you move to IVF and you make the egg and the sperm meet in a dish, the effect of endometriosis seems not to be that great … But there is a big but, and the big but is that a lot of women have endometriosis, and they will also have another condition. We call it the sister condition, and that's adenomyosis.

We see that endometriosis with adenomyosis has quite a significant adverse impact on women's fertility, even in the setting of IVF. So we know that they're less likely to achieve a pregnancy when we've done an embryo transfer, and sadly, if they have achieved the pregnancy, then they're quite a bit more likely to miscarry. So, for an IVF specialist, the focus is usually more on the adenomyosis than the endometriosis.

Asked when chances of pregnancy are highest, he says:

Fertility optimisation is still around 27 for fertility, and then it starts going downhill from there. We find the optimal egg quality between 25 and 30. Young women's eggs will improve towards the mid-20s; after 30, there is a very shallow decline until 35. Then, it starts to accelerate a little bit more. And then after 40, yes, between 40 and 45, you're dropping off a cliff.

Dr Samantha Mooney on treatment options

Dr Mooney is a highly skilled obstetrician, gynaecologist and fertility doctor with specialist training in minimally invasive surgical techniques. Dr Mooney specialises in endometriosis and adenomyosis and provides specialised care at Mercy Hospital for Women, Epworth Healthcare, Warringal Hospital and Genea Fertility. She is also a researcher who has investigated the impact of pre-pregnancy surgical treatment of endometriosis on future obstetric outcomes and evidence for multidisciplinary care in pelvic pain and endometriosis. I asked her about fertility, the process of egg retrieval and how it affects women+ with endo.

Often, the 18-year-old comes to my room with their mum, and she [the mum] wants to know about her daughter's future fertility. The 18-year-old doesn't want to know anything about it (yet!) but they want help with their pain. However, when a 30-year-old comes to my room often they really want to know about their fertility, alongside treatment of any other symptoms. Sometimes, they aren't attending with any pain symptoms associated with endometriosis, but are facing the challenges of infertility.

If the patient is concerned about a future pregnancy or I am aware there may be an issue with their egg reserve, we can arrange egg retrieval and freeze these eggs for potential future use. We used to freeze either eggs or ovary tissue, but techniques weren't as successful. We can now vitrify eggs ("snap freeze"). With this technology, egg freezing—which in essence involves the first half of an IVF cycle—has become much more mainstream. We take mature eggs and freeze them, which differs from harvesting ovary tissue where the eggs are still immature. If the patient has fertility issues in the future, the eggs can then be thawed, and fertilised using ICSI.

Patients with endometriosis and persistent pelvic pain, have got the added stress of being in a fertility cycle, the social stresses, and the juggling work, on top of their usual symptoms. I'm doing a procedure where I stick a needle through the tissues of the vagina, potentially irritating the muscles of the pelvic floor to collect those eggs; rather than ovulating one follicle, you've got the fluid potentially from multiple follicles leaking out into the pelvis, a little bit of blood as well, which is what happens with ovulation. However, ovulation itself is very painful for some patients.

Even though I've aspirated all those eggs out, the ovaries remain enlarged for several weeks. Even in a 'normal' IVF cycle, even for someone who conceives. We often see these 'IVF ovaries' until they're eight weeks' or 10 weeks' pregnant.

I always try to manage the patient's expectations. I explain that this might be a sensitising event for someone who has complex pelvic pain, and I make sure they've got their multidisciplinary team around them, and encourage them to avoid foods or stressors that exacerbate their symptoms. I encourage them to take adequate time off work to recover.

I strongly believe in multidisciplinary care. I make sure their physiotherapist and pain specialist are aware, and if they've got another gynaecologist, they know of any procedures and the approach I have taken. I also try to manage the expectations of patients and their caregivers. They may have spoken to friends who've had an IVF cycle and sailed through it without problems.

However, those with endometriosis and adenomyosis have a higher sensitisation to hormones, to medical procedures and pain throughout their pelvis.

Also, we are mindful that ovarian hyperstimulation syndrome [OHSS; when the ovaries have an exaggerated response to the hormones and swell and become painful, and the patient can have swelling or excess fluid in their abdomen and sometimes lungs] probably affects half to 1 per cent of patients undergoing FSH stimulation. IVF nursing staff across all clinics call patients on the first day. There's 24-7 access to discuss if there are symptoms. Patients are also advised to present their concerns about symptoms to their nearest emergency department. OHSS is painful, but some patients will not report it as pain; they feel incredibly bloated and incredibly heavy.

It is a privilege to treat and care for endo warriors, and I do my best to manage their expectations for pain, other symptom relief and fertility.

When IVF has a happy ending: Alicia's story

Alicia is my niece, my sister's eldest daughter, whose husband is in the military. As a result, the family have lived interstate and overseas for decades. It was confronting to see Alicia so debilitated by pain, which we put down to a training mishap and fibromyalgia.

It never occurred to us that it could be endometriosis; her symptoms were different to those my daughter Brianna experienced. I am extremely grateful to Professor Louise Hull and feel blessed to have been in Adelaide when Alicia had IVF egg retrieval, to learn about her positive pregnancy, and to accompany Alicia for the final ultrasound before having the opportunity to meet my perfect great-niece. Alicia talks about her fertility and endo journey and how it was all worth it in the end.

For nine years, I kept a note titled 'symptoms' on my phone:

'fluctuating appetite, nausea, painful cramps before and during period, light-headedness, bloating, hot flushes, night sweats, recurring mouth ulcers, irregular and heavy bleeding (10 days of bleeding), swollen armpit lymph nodes, sore/stiff joints, lethargy, headaches first thing in the morning, constant lower back pain (worse before period), weird heartbeat, chest pain'.

Whenever I went to a new GP every year or so due to regular interstate and international moves, I would read out my list. Without fail, I would be sent off for blood tests just to be told I was healthy besides sporadic anaemia, and that I was most likely just stressed and overthinking.

I remember one GP telling me that, as an 18-year-old, they believed I had convinced myself that I was sick and my ailments were psychosomatic. I was referred, at one point, to a rheumatologist who, within five minutes of a telehealth call, diagnosed me with fibromyalgia, prescribed amitriptyline and told me to follow-up in six months.

I knew something wasn't right. Surely, it was more than fibromyalgia. Having periods that cause you to throw up and be curled up in pain for days was not normal, but I thought they were. For nine years, I thought I was just being dramatic. It became easier to suffer silently than to be ignored.

I saw a gynaecologist for the first time when I was 23, and only after I had done the research and booked a GP appointment solely to obtain a referral to the OBGYN of my choice.

I cannot believe I was never referred to a gynaecologist based on my symptoms. This gynaecologist said my ultrasound looked 'messy' and that my best chance to have children was to start trying now.

Over the next two years, my husband and I experienced the grief and trauma that come with four miscarriages and an interstitial ectopic pregnancy. I worked through all the miscarriages. I remember that each time I started bleeding, I was at work, and by the third, I thought, 'Well, there it is'. Pregnancy loss had become my reality, my expectation. After my ectopic pregnancy, I had to wait three months before trying again, and when the OBGYN gave me the green light, I remember saying, 'I have to travel for work next month and don't have time for a miscarriage'—as soon as the words came out of my mouth, I knew I couldn't keep putting my body, mind and spirit through it, so we stopped trying.

After moving interstate for my husband's job, I researched fertility specialists in Adelaide, requested a referral from my GP in ACT and, to my luck, was in with the most amazing specialist weeks after arriving in South Australia.

At my first appointment, this specialist said she was very confident I had endometriosis based on my symptoms, and she wanted to book me in for a laparoscopy and hysteroscopy in the coming weeks. I remember feeling like I was going to burst with excitement. Finally, I was seen and heard. I wasn't dismissed and was told that tracking my symptoms was smart and helpful.

I had heard of endometriosis as my cousin had been diagnosed years prior and had several excisions; however, I knew very little about it. Naturally, I googled it as soon as I got home that day and, when I read the symptoms, it was like reading the list I had on my phone.

I called my cousin, who walked me through what the operation and recovery may be like. She even sent me a care package that significantly helped during my recovery: a wheat heat pack, fluffy bed socks, a button-down nighty, extra op-site dressings, and Coloxyl [a stool softener].

After my operation, my specialist told me she had removed the endometriosis she could find, my left fallopian tube was significantly damaged from the ectopic pregnancy and was permanently blocked, and I had polycystic ovaries. I finally had *answers; I could feel the weight of nine years of pain and the constant battle to be heard lifted off my shoulders. Everything I felt wasn't just in my head, I was finally validated.*

Shortly after my laparoscopic operation, my husband and I decided we wanted to try IVF. We were very blessed to fall pregnant on our first round with the help of progesterone and a whole lot of luck. I ensured I followed the suggestions/superstitions I had picked up from the various IVF communities I trailed. Acupuncture directly before and after my frozen embryo transfer, keeping my feet warm for 48 hours, eating a serving of Maccas fries (more of a good luck gesture) and drinking pomegranate juice.

I had absolutely zero symptoms leading up to my Beta HCG test [blood test for pregnancy]. I decided to take a home pregnancy test the night before my blood test so I could mentally prepare myself and I could find out myself rather than being told over the phone.

After the longest five minutes of my life, my husband and I looked at the two lines together. You would expect a reaction of overwhelming joy; however, unexpectedly, my stomach immediately dropped and panic set in as I entered fight or flight mode. Seeing those two lines took me back to the only reality I knew: loss.

After I finally accepted that this was happening, which, believe me, took a while, I had the most beautiful pregnancy. As I write this, my beautiful baby girl is sleeping soundly beside me in her bassinet. Too often, with endo comes infertility or recurring pregnancy loss, but with timely diagnosis and intervention can come hope.

Dealing with the tough stuff

Discussing having a family of your own can be difficult for you and your partner; you may not be on the same timeline, particularly if you have endometriosis, adenomyosis or PCOS and know it may not be as easy as tracking ovulation and having sex.

Deciding to try for a baby is also an emotional roller-coaster, with performance anxiety killing the mood and the weight of expectation when your period is due. When your period arrives, it can prompt a grief response and make you feel like you've failed.

It is common for couples to share feelings of anxiety, fear, sadness, worthlessness, resentment and lash out with blame. All of these emotions can make any existing relationship issues worse.

Counselling before starting the pregnancy journey can help air issues, fears and concerns and manage unhelpful responses and difficult behaviours. Fertility clinics also offer counselling to confront any issues; let you know what to expect, emotionally as well as hormonally; and to support you when a cycle doesn't result in eggs, embryos aren't viable or transfers don't result in pregnancy.

In around 70 per cent of cases, endometriosis and adenomyosis don't result in infertility.

For those who do seek IVF treatment, some studies show there are lower pregnancy rates for those with endo and adeno than those with other infertility diagnoses. Another study showed that surgically treated endometriosis resulted in higher live births than those cases that were untreated.

It is also important to be aware of premature menopause among women+ with endometriosis, and that this may affect your fertility. If you have been on hormone treatment, it can be hard to track periods or you may not have any. As we discussed, egg reserves can be lower due to lesions, adhesions and surgery. Jean Hailes has a checklist for perimenopause and menopause to help you recognise Premature Ovarian Insufficiency.

Unfortunately, pregnancy and birth rates are reported to be even lower for adenomyosis compared with endometriosis. The miscarriage and stillbirth (after 20 weeks) rates are higher than those without this condition because the endometriosis cells, like the lining on the inside of your uterus, are also in the muscle wall of your uterus and can cause adhesions. Studies suggest that about one in five women+ have this condition. For those living with adenomyosis, where the embryo lands is important. Please seek support and resources through the wonderful team at Pink Elephants (pinkelephants.org.au).

When IVF doesn't end as hoped: Ellie's story

We first met Ellie Angel-Mobbs, an award-winning radio announcer and advocate for endo, adeno and infertility, back in Chapter 4. Ellie has endured five rounds of IVF and has now accepted that she won't have a baby of her own.

I was 25 when I met Jamie, and that's when I got sick with the endo. Within the first six months of our dating, we were sitting in a gynaecologist's rooms. The doctor looked at us and said, 'Ellie, it seems like you've got endometriosis. You two should go off and have a baby', and I remember looking at Jamie going, my God, we've just started dating.

What kind of conversation is this to have with this new person? I knew then and there that he was my forever person, but still, that's the biggest test to go through when they throw those curve balls out like that. For me, as a young thing, to hear this from this male professional who was fantastic but didn't have the greatest bedside manner, and to be told, go and have a baby — the words were like, 'Hey, go and boil the kettle and make a cup of tea', that's how easy it is to fall pregnant.

At 25, my plans didn't include a baby; I wanted to live my best life, have fun and travel. I told myself, 'Babies can wait; I'll be right'. I was not thinking things through as to how hard it would be, especially for someone like me who then goes on to be diagnosed with adenomyosis, a damaged uterus and stage 4 endo.

We had problems falling pregnant, and the five rounds of IVF were hard. I don't think anyone could ever prepare you for IVF, no matter how many books, podcasts or chats you have — you're entering into this whole new world where you don't know what will be around the corner.

By the fifth round, the doctor told me I needed to see a kidney specialist; stop the drugs, stop everything because I now had stage 3 kidney issues. It was underlying the sepsis, which I ended up contracting twice. I couldn't tolerate the IVF drugs.

The kidney doctor looked me squarely in the eye and said, if you fall pregnant, either you'll die, or the baby will die.

As a result, we've closed the book on me becoming a mum, and I'm the crazy dog lady and the awesome auntie. My husband is a keeper. He's an absolute treasure. I am so lucky to have found him. He had two kids from a previous marriage, I'm a stepmom. I get to be a mother in that aspect, but Jamie constantly says to me all the time when he sees me with my nephews, and he sees me with other children, and says the world missed out on that.

I struggle around newborn kids, especially in an office environment. Pregnancy announcements upset me, and I've let the management know, 'Please, can you excuse me if there is a pregnancy announcement? I don't want to be there when you make it.' My beautiful team at Southern Cross Austereo (SCA) understand where I'm coming from and know where I have been. I have little security blankets around me to ensure I avoid triggers.

I am now planning for the hysterectomy the gynaecologist told me I would eventually need back when I was in my mid-twenties. I got to almost 40. I've always had that thought in the back of my mind, knowing Mum needed it and that her sisters had similar scenarios. I'm looking at timing; how long will I need off from work? Who knows what they're going to find in there this time? I've been warned that I may need a colorectal surgeon at the same time.

I'm excited at the thought that a hysterectomy might help relieve the pain. Still, at the end of the day, it is not going to cure my endometriosis, but it may bring relief for the pain which I do suffer from.

I wish I'd seen a specialist earlier and not procrastinated and put it off. I just dismissed my symptoms as being normal, and that period pain was just something that we would put up with because that's what I got taught at school. Despite knowing Mum had endometriosis, which can cause this debilitating pain, I didn't put two and two together.

I cancelled multiple endo related medical appointments just because I was like, 'Nah, I'll be right, I'm too busy. I've got a social life. See ya, medical problems. I'll worry about that when I'm older.' When you're in your early twenties, you don't realise that you have that one body and that you really should be putting as much love and care into it as possible and not going out and, you know, partying the night away.

Fertility is fleeting. Look after yours.

Be aware

Pink Elephants Support Network was founded by Samantha Payne, an endo warrior also living with adeno, after she experienced the heartache of multiple miscarriages. Visit pinkelephants.org.au for information and support.

Be prepared

Couples counselling can help to air your thoughts, dreams, concerns and fears. IVF services offer specific counselling around fertility, cycle failures and pregnancy loss.

CHAPTER 9

Multidisciplinary care

The biomedical approach studies the human body in health and disease. It seeks to identify and treat specific physical causes of pain, such as infections, inflammation or structural abnormalities. Treatments typically include medications (e.g. antibiotics, anti-inflammatory drugs, pain relievers), surgical interventions and physical therapies aimed at correcting or alleviating the identified physical issues.

This approach often overlooks the psychological and social dimensions of pain. It may not fully address the complexity of chronic pain conditions, which can persist even when no clear physical cause is found or after the physical issue has been treated.

Biopsychosocial approaches

The biopsychosocial approach, proposed by George Engel in 1977, considers the interplay between biological, psychological and social factors. It views pain as a complex, multifaceted experience influenced by a combination of these factors This involves a comprehensive treatment plan that addresses:

- Biological factors: Similar to the biomedical approach, it includes medications and physical therapies.
- Psychological factors: Interventions may include cognitive behavioural therapy, stress management and addressing mental health issues, such as anxiety and depression.

- Social factors: It considers the patient's social environment, relationships, work situation and overall lifestyle. Interventions might include social support, counselling and lifestyle modifications.

The biopsychosocial model is more holistic and patient-centred. It aims to improve overall quality of life by addressing all aspects of the patient's experience. This approach is particularly effective for chronic (recurring) conditions like chronic or persistent pelvic pain, where pain persists despite the absence of clear physical pathology.

In practice, this model requires a multidisciplinary team, including healthcare providers from various fields, such as medicine, psychology, physiotherapy and social work. This team collaborates to create a personalised treatment plan for the patient.

Changing the narrative: Julia's story

The Julia Argyrou Endometriosis Centre at Epworth (JAECE) in Melbourne was established in 2022 with a philanthropic gift from the Argyrou family and other donors. Its focus is on research and person-centred integrated care, aiming to 'increase healthcare provider and community awareness of endometriosis and empower patients to act by developing and providing access to improved models of care while seeking new understanding of prevention, diagnosis, and treatment of endometriosis'.

I am privileged to count Julia as a close friend. When we share long walks together, endometriosis is always the 'third wheel', with Julia's pain her constant companion.

Julia was diagnosed at age 21, after seven years of having her pain dismissed. She was told that her excruciating pain was nothing more than constipation and was prescribed laxatives. Like many women+, she had her appendix removed — it was perfectly healthy and her pain continued unabated.

Her husband Michael has been by her side for 16 operations to treat endometriosis infiltration of her ovaries, kidneys, uterus, fallopian tubes, bowel, cervix, intestines, diagram and rectum — she also has adenomyosis. But wait, there's more! Endometriosis has affected her central nervous system and leg nerves.

Miraculously, Julia has four children, all in their twenties. She worries about her three girls and the genetic link for future generations.

She says, 'My wish is to not only find a cure but to make others' experiences with endo very different from mine'. Julia, supported by Michael, refused to accept that her suffering was merely 'normal' menstrual pain, as many doctors had suggested in the past. Julia's journey became a quest for answers, for a solution that would bring relief to herself and others.

Imagine, if you will, what it's like to live in a body where even the simplest actions can trigger excruciating pain. Every step I take, every breath I draw, every decision I make is dictated by the pain that courses through me. It dominates my thoughts, colours my emotions and steals precious moments I can never regain.

Endometriosis is an invisible illness. From the outside, I may appear fine, but inside, my body is engaged in a constant struggle, attacking itself and causing incomprehensible pain. It's a battle that leaves me feeling isolated, misunderstood and trapped within a body that does not feel like my own.

The suffering doesn't end there. Endometriosis takes a toll not only physically but also mentally and emotionally. It's a constant juggling act between managing pain, navigating countless doctors' appointments, enduring invasive procedures, and dealing with the emotional implications of fertility challenges. It's a burden that weighs heavily on my spirit, threatening to rob me of the joy and optimism that should define my life.

Together, we can change the narrative surrounding endometriosis. We can build a world where women like me don't have to endure the daily torment that comes with this condition. By standing together, we can create a future where our voices are heard, our suffering is acknowledged and our pain is no longer invisible.

I share my story with you not to invoke pity but to inspire empathy and understanding. I want you to truly grasp the profound impact that endometriosis has on the lives of millions of women around the world. We need your support, understanding and advocacy to make a difference.

By raising our collective voices, we can push for change. We can demand better treatments, more research funding, and improved healthcare practices for women living with endometriosis. Let us not rest until our pain is acknowledged, our experiences validated and our needs met.

To the medical community, I implore you to listen to us, to take our concerns seriously, and to work towards more effective treatments and, ultimately, a cure. To researchers and scientists, we need your unwavering dedication to unravelling the mysteries of this complex condition.

Stephanie O'Kane on supporting patients' varied needs

Stephanie, one of the endometriosis nurse coordinators at the Julia Argyrou Endometriosis Centre at Epworth in Melbourne, chose to dedicate herself to nursing women's health and like many of us, endo found her. She is committed to supporting endo warriors those affected by endometriosis to live well with the life-defining disease. By the time the patient is in front of her, they've already had a round-the-world trip with the medical sector. She hears patients say, 'It feels like we're just going around in circles about the same things'.

It's not fun for a person to present to ED, to come into the GP and talk about their pain and quality of life. That's not something that people enjoy generally. If they make those steps and that conscious effort to come to you, as a medical practitioner, the very least we can do is be a validating space and fully, fully listen and not just hear what we think we want to hear but hear what they're saying. I also think what goes hand in hand with that is knowing what we should be listening for because it's one thing to listen well, however, suppose you're not picking up on certain markers. In that case, you may not signpost them correctly just because you weren't aware of endometriosis symptoms.

She hopes more school nurses, triage and clinic nurses, and doctors are making an effort to 'keep up to date with chronic pelvic pain ... with the pain science behind it'

There's growing recognition that we see endometriosis now as a chronic systemic condition. A disease that affects multiple systems within the body. It's not just a sole disease of the pelvis anymore. We're moving away from that ideology.

When we acknowledge all the different body systems that endometriosis can affect, we need a lot of different disciplines ... to be involved throughout someone's life to achieve appropriate care.

Stephanie recognises that, while all her patients wish to be well and pain free, what they want from their lives is different and this can shape the way she approaches her care and her recommendations for their future care.

It's really important to start the conversation with the patient about quality of life and what a person wants their life to look like. You can't presume. Once we've narrowed down their goals, we can start to put in place who might be best equipped to get them to where they want to be.

It is helpful when patients track symptoms and bring previous tests and scans to medical appointments. As a nurse, I focus on the complete history of the patient. We want to know where you're at in life right now. What is your most impactful symptom? And what do you need from us? It is about two-way communication. What I think is best for you might not be what you think is best.

For example, fertility discussions are really important. Sometimes I feel like fertility isn't talked about enough, but then sometimes I feel like it's a little bit oversaturated, where people can come away and feel that they weren't seen as a person; they were seen as their ability to conceive and procreate. I always like to ask people, 'What are your thoughts about fertility?' I'm asking this question with absolutely no agenda. It's just helpful for me to know so that when you do go on to see another clinician, I can let them know patient X is concerned about fertility, would like to conceive in the next one to two years, or is not concerned about their fertility, not wanting to have a pregnancy. In these conversations, there's no wrong or right answer. It is my job to triage what they need, what's most important versus what's not really important to them.

I aim to reassure patients that I am here to tailor-make a treatment plan for them. I like to know what you have tried in the past. What hasn't worked? And if it hasn't worked, were there any negative symptoms? We want to know all these things so there's a sense that you, as a patient, won't go round and round in circles with your treatment plan.

When seeking support for endometriosis and chronic pain, the journey can be overwhelming. Stephanie emphasises the benefits of utilising your support group and the tools you have at hand.

Patients should be aware that it's okay to bring an advocate with you if you have someone like a family member or a friend and you feel more comfortable. A second set of ears is always welcome. I think, especially when you leave that appointment, having someone to debrief with is a really empowering tool.

Know that it's not rude to take notes during your consultation to prompt you to ask other questions.

We also know that the endometriosis enigma often changes symptoms from cycle to cycle, from flare-up to flare-up. Someone might not have any troublesome symptoms for six months, and then they go down, as the old saying goes, like spuds. And it's important to recognise that you need a toolkit of different options.

Validation is really important, and I think it's okay for both the patient and the clinician to admit that they don't have all the answers. I think that speaks more, and having someone who's transparent with you is really, really important because honesty and rawness go a long way in establishing rapport.

Often, the first consultation is emotionally heavy, and patients shouldn't feel uncomfortable about that. It may be the first time that they've been given space to talk about what they need to and be believed.

But my hope is that through those appointments, there's a little glimmer of hope of some things to hold on to, so they feel 'I've really been heard this time and I'm feeling a bit more positive about what might come next.'

While we are there for informal emotional support, we do highlight that we, as endo nurse coordinators, are not mental health professionals. We suggest options for psychological support and how to get a mental health care plan from the GP.

Support can look different to different people. Sometimes, it's friends or family, but sometimes, people choose to look outside their circle, and joining support groups with others is powerful. Getting a young person to journal, or outside and doing something they love is a great example of powerful forms of self-care.

Receiving support from an understanding healthcare professional is the first step to optimal management of symptoms and pain. Consulting with an endo nurse, like Stephanie, can extend to beyond physical symptoms and whole-of-life approaches to managing the physical and psychological impacts of endo.

One aspect of endometriosis is the difficulty of predicting when symptoms will hit. If you're making plans and you're someone that may be prone to flares that relate to pain, you could say something as simple as, 'Right now, that sounds so amazing and I'd be happy to be there, but please just be mindful that I may have to cancel at the last minute. It's not my intention, but it may happen.' It is worth cultivating a network around you that would be accepting of that answer and wouldn't challenge you on that.

I have a general conversation about how nutrition can have a positive impact and can enhance wellbeing from a broader perspective. There is no leading gold standard at the moment when it comes to endometriosis nutrition. We can't say one diet is better, but we can say, 'Have you tried this? Would you be willing to try this? Is this going to be the case? Do you have the mental effort to make these changes right now?' And for some people, it is very achievable and, anecdotally, they will see positive results. But again, it's just showing people the different options to treat a chronic condition.

Starting down the endo care journey is overwhelming. If you've gone down the Doctor Google rabbit hole, you will have been confronted with a staggering amount of information and recommendations. This is where it helps to have an experienced health professional in your corner to cut through the noise.

We don't want to make care feel like a burden. We want it to be achievable. If you tell a patient to go away and do all of these things and they feel overwhelmed, it's likely that they may not do any of it because it all becomes really difficult. We want that bite-sized care that they feel that they can achieve themselves but not give away too much of their energy in doing so.

The financial burden of endometriosis and other chronic conditions is also overwhelming. So, wherever we can direct to resources that will not cost out of pocket, it is important to share those resources, especially the evidence-based and free ones you can find on the JAECE website, EndoZone, and Jean Hailes for Women's Health websites.

AT JAECE, we have regular webinars, and you can find the past ones on the website. You need to subscribe to webinar updates, then you'll be sent the link before they go live.

Telehealth communications are so important to our chronic cohort, and we want to make access easy. We want to bring things into their home so that they do not have to use energy. It's exhausting, and there are enough things to be exhausted about already.

Particularly in the winter, it's just another added layer of discomfort getting out to a medical appointment.

If you can be at home with your jammies on, with your heat pack under your jammies, and if you don't want the camera on, that's fine. We'll get everything we need for our purposes.

Allied health

Allied health practitioners are university qualified and provide treatment aimed at preventing, diagnosing and treating conditions and illnesses. They include physiotherapy, osteopathy, exercise physiologists, psychology, pharmacy, dietitians and nutritionists.

Pelvic physiotherapy

We might not get you rolling on the pelvic floor laughing, but let's get the femur to introduce some humur so you can make the hip joint happy.

Growing up, I attended a Brigandine Catholic girls' school, which had real nuns, including Sister Cecilia—try saying that with a lisp—who told us to strengthen our pelvic floor to prevent weeing away from the toilet. I would religiously do Kegel exercises, especially in the car, visualising sitting on a marble and lifting it, holding it tightly for three seconds, then relaxing.

However, for those living with endometriosis and pelvic pain, tightening isn't the answer—relaxing is. In endometriosis, the pelvic floor can become rigid. Mobility exercises, manual therapy and teaching strategies help in managing pain and alleviating tension and nerve sensitivity. Having a functional pelvic floor helps with bladder control and weeing, bowel pain and pooing, improves libido, arousal and reduces pain during sex.

Professor Luk Rombauts (who we met in Chapter 8) is a big believer in pelvic physiotherapy and says you need to get onto pelvic floor dysfunction early:

> We know physiotherapy, yoga, Pilates and pelvic floor physio exercises help the pain. Patients would like to have a baby, but the pain has now gotten so bad that that has to become the priority, and they are concerned about stopping treatment to get pregnant. Some are taking so many different painkillers, often like having a whole cocktail every day, and someone has to sort it out.
>
> The pelvic floor physiotherapists in my practice have been extremely helpful. I think it's often overlooked how the pain can originate in the uterus or around the uterus. Still, because people have been coping so much with chronic pain, their pelvic floor becomes so dysfunctional that they constantly find that they've got cramping in those muscles and spasms. Surgery will not fix that. You need pain education ... make sure they understand what pain is, where it originates from, when it becomes acute, when it goes from acute to chronic, and when it goes from peripheral to central pain. And having that better understanding and realistic expectations

Multidisciplinary care **115**

of what an interdisciplinary or multidisciplinary approach can bring will be extremely beneficial for the patient managing all of the symptoms.

Ellie Angel-Mobbs says:

I have seen a pelvic physio, and they said that my pelvic floor was like a rock, and I just need to relax. I urge others with endo to go and get their pelvic floor checked out because it affects bladder control, bowel control and all of the things that cause pain as well.

Akaiti James on her approach to holistic care

Akaiti is an endo warrior who has a Bachelor of Biomedical Science with first-class honours from the University of Western Australia. She has a double degree in immunology, microbiology pathology, and laboratory medicine and, while completing a medical degree, she is doing a part-time PhD in endometriosis. She is the president of Endometriosis WA.

She remembers feeling 'sore' from when she got her first period around the age of 13. She too experienced quite the journey to diagnosis (finally at the age of 27), including having her (healthy) appendix removed when doctors thought it was the source of her pain. Even after surgery:

My symptoms continued. I thought I might have endometriosis after doing a lot of 'Doctor Googling'. The GP said to me, 'No, this won't be endometriosis' because I was saying that I was having pain at ovulation time.

Being 27, I was quite insistent on being able to advocate for myself a bit more than someone a lot younger would probably feel comfortable doing. I asked for a referral to a specialist, and I asked for one with Australasian Gynaecological Endoscopy (AGES) certification.

After the laparoscopic surgery, I definitely saw an improvement in my endometriosis symptoms, but still have residual kind of chronic pain issues from what we call central sensitisation, which is the dysregulation of pain, the pain signals and your brain's recognition of pain signals that occurs from living with pain for so long.

Growing up, Akaiti thought her pain was 'normal'. 'My mum probably had endometriosis, she'd always be talking about her periods being sore, and we just got on with it.' For Akaiti, the pain never really goes away.

> You learn to manage it, which I guess I'm fortunate in that I have, you know, been able to manage it mostly through ovulation suppression, so, continuously taking an OCP hormone pill. It took me a while to find one that worked for me, but it did in the end. Unfortunately, it's not on the PBS. I am paying a fair bit for it, which can be difficult because having endometriosis is expensive and I've been a student for a while now.
>
> The cost of managing endometriosis is estimated at around $3900 per year by the AIHW [Australian Institute of Health and Welfare]. Still, once you factor in medication, scans, GP appointments, specialist appointments, pain medications and period items if you're ovulating, it is even higher, particularly with laparoscopic surgery.
>
> Endometriosis is also affecting life choices. I am currently a third-year medical student, but surgery is a very physical job. It's a lot of standing, standing in one position, long hours, and different work schedules. Night shift can exacerbate chronic pain.

For some women+, pelvic physiotherapy can be a game changer.

> When you're in pain, especially severe pain, you just disconnect. Pelvic physio made a huge difference for me. It involves learning to reconnect with your body. It is very holistic. They ask you when you go to your appointment, 'How's your pain?' 'How are your bowels?' 'How's your bladder?' Because even in Western medicine, we tend to specialise in everything and take different specialties and different body areas. Pelvic health services are very poor in rural and regional areas. We have one of our volunteers who lives in Albany, which is about a five-hour drive from Perth. She drives to Perth monthly for her pelvic physio appointment.

There is a great WA-based physio app and a group called Matilda (matilda.health) that provides support for people with endometriosis. The services can be accessed through the phone app anywhere in Australia.

For self-care, Akaiti says:

> *Magnesium with Epsom salts have been recommended, and that's been a big help for me. Diet helps. I would love to say I have a perfect diet, but I don't. Anti-inflammatory foods, eating well, a balanced diet, a Mediterranean diet, as they call it, which is so hard when you're very busy, maintaining good sleep hygiene, getting enough sleep — that's crucial for managing pain. Alcohol will flare me up.*
>
> *Take advantage of your chronic condition management plans from your GP, which will give you sessions with two or three different allied health specialists.*
>
> *I'm not running anymore, which is a shame. You can get exercise physiologists or physiotherapists to help you work out what is good for you, something that's not going to flare your pelvic floor and is providing you with the exercise that you need. And with those plans, you can get dietitians, who then can help you if you're not managing with recipes. ChatGPT is great for that, by the way. I say, 'I don't like tomato and salad, I don't like tuna.' I put a maximum preparation time of 15 minutes, and it'll spit out a whole meal plan for you with recipes. Work smarter, I say, and get inspiration to eat something quick and healthy.*

Rachel Andrew with the lowdown on physio below the belt

Vagenius is an approved national training provider for the doctors at the RANZCOG, RACGP and ACRRM, and it is approved as evidence-based for EndoZone.

Rachel, co-founder of Vagenius, is an Australian Physiotherapy Association continence and women+'s health physiotherapist with a BSc in physiotherapy, a clinical master of women+'s health, and a certificate in conservative management of prolapse.

A patient may be referred to a pelvic physiotherapist by their GP, gynaecologist or other allied health practitioner. You don't actually need a referral to see a physiotherapist, even one specialising in pelvic pain. Rachel says, regardless of how you come to her, she'll ask 'lots of questions, and that'll include bladder and bowel history, history of your periods, if you've had any births or any pregnancies at all, and your general health'.

Rachel looks at the whole person dealing with the pain.

Regardless of what I like to call the pain's name — in this case, it may be endometriosis or adenomyosis. We also know there are so many comorbidities; for many with endo and adeno, the pain isn't just pelvic, it affects the whole body. I ask them about their history of depression or anxiety and how they manage that. I'll delve into their personal situation. Do they have support at home? Do they have pets that they love? Do they have children?

I'll start talking about some specific things, like sexual health. Is sex fun and pleasurable? Not all people know that it should be fun and pleasurable for everyone.

We'll talk about hobbies. If someone has a long history of dancing, horse riding, or snowboarding, those are typical ones that can be linked with pelvic floor tension, tailbone injuries, and deep hip or lower back pain. Usually, these things can be treated and get better.

Women with endo and back pain don't get better. I ask them in detail about their pain, and if they have bladder pain, for example, I'll say that when you're emptying, when your bladder's full, do you get cramps after you empty? Can you make it through a meeting or a movie before needing a wee?

Is it low-down entry urethral pain or is it lower tummy pain? If it's lower tummy pain, then that's often a different part of the pelvic floor than urethral pain, and we treat them differently.

The same goes for the bowel. Are you having general abdominal pain or bloating? Do you get much wind? Do you get left-sided or right-sided pain? Do you get pain when you poo? Do you get pain afterwards? Is your bowel fluctuating? I'll also ask about fatigue as part of general health.

I will ask about other conditions, especially if they've been living with pain for a long time. Have they been diagnosed with fibromyalgia, chronic fatigue, bladder pain syndrome or irritable bowel? These can be related to endometriosis and adenomyosis. I try to tease out in the general health whether they've got other things like thyroid issues or if they've ever had any pelvic or abdominal surgery, and I ask about medications they're taking for their pain. Sometimes hormonal treatments, along with supplements like iron, can also affect pain, and analgesics can affect the bowel and toileting.

I particularly want to know if they are taking opioids — already part of my goal is to try and get them off the opioids, to support them in getting their pain under control so that they have space to work on that deep dependence with their doctor. There can be opioid-induced myalgia, which is muscle pain within six weeks of use, which is worrying. Codeine can give you constipation, you can get oesophageal reflux. When I write back to their doctor, I'll try and ask them to do a medication review so we can kind of work together to look at non-medication options for pain relief.

Sex is a huge part of what we do for women with endo because, often, women with endo do not have pleasurable sex, and that can be a physical reason. I mean, it's also mental, like if you're not having sex that you enjoy, no-one wants to do it. One in four women will have pain with sex, and one in ten men at some time in their life. If you have a male partner and you ask them what it would feel like to get an erection with their penis in a vice, that's like you can get clitoral pain with arousal. The same muscles that wrap around the bladder and the bowel and are attached to the tailbone are the muscles of sex, and they go behind the clitoris. They have to relax and open as you get aroused. However, arousal for women is so different.

I want to hear what their pain is stopping them from doing and how their pain makes them feel about themselves because there's a real spectrum. Some people are like, 'Oh, it's annoying me. I want to sort it out'. For others who've been living with endo for a long time and maybe have sought help for ten or 15 years, it's really become a deep part of themselves. They are negative, with poor self-image. They think they are weaker than other people or lazier; there are a lot of bad personal associations between you and your sense of self.

Rachel says that diet can make a difference to the inflammation caused by endo.

For those who have a name for their pain and are feeling helpless to do anything to minimise the impact of endometriosis, I encourage them to look at their diet. I encourage them to look at an anti-inflammatory approach — we know endo is an inflammatory condition — to cut out things like gluten or milk and see if they feel better, and encourage them to see a good a naturopath, nutritionist. I direct them to EndoZone or Pelvic Pain Foundation of Australia for information on managing symptoms.

There are also tools that a physiotherapist can recommend to ease pain.

For many with pelvic pain, even with endo, I can show them how to use a wand for a bit of pelvic floor manual therapy. The magic wand is a curved device. You can buy it from the physiotherapist or through the Pelvic Pain Foundation of Australia. They come in a few different shapes and sizes and are in an S shape. The pelvic floor muscles are like a deep bowl, so as you go into the vagina and, if people are curious, you can put your finger in and feel a lot of this. They can treat themselves well, and they're happy.

A TENS [transcutaneous electrical nerve stimulation] machine can be a really great device, and there are some really good ones out on the market now that are designed for women with endo. They really work by almost distracting your nerve supply and giving you control over what's happening. They give your brain a signal that your brain thinks is pain, but you don't feel it as pain.

Multidisciplinary, allied and integrative health are holistic because they treat the whole person. I urge other health practitioners to listen for phrases like pulling pain, abdominal pain, bloating and profound pain with sex to make a referral to a gynaecologist.

Be aware

It is really important that we talk about relaxing, not only strengthening the pelvic floor. Physiotherapy is often covered by private health insurance, if you have it. Many women+'s hospitals also offer it in the public health system.

Be prepared

Vagenius pelvic exercises for endo is in the resources.

Weight training is so important, especially if you've been on hormone medications. We know that lifting weights two times a week is crucial for bone density, mood and balance.

Acupuncture for endo

Acupuncture is fabulous because, when we think about endo as a neuro-inflammatory disease, acupuncture can be beneficial in calming the nervous system. It is increasingly being explored as a complementary treatment for endometriosis, particularly for alleviating associated pelvic pain. Research suggests that acupuncture can provide clinically significant improvements in pain management and overall quality of life.

The insertion of needles stimulates nerve receptors, which can activate the body's natural pain-relieving mechanisms, including the release of endorphins and modulation of pain pathways in the central nervous system. Research indicates that acupuncture can lower levels of inflammatory markers such as CA-125, which is often elevated in those with endometriosis. This reduction may help alleviate symptoms by decreasing inflammation in affected tissues.

Ellie Angel-Mobbs says:

> I love acupuncture. It is my favourite thing. I love, love, love, love, love it. I highly recommend that anyone do it. I've done it for endo, I did it when I was doing IVF rounds. I was in there three times a week when we were doing the rounds... That was fantastic. I take magnesium and daily supplements, vitamin D, all of those things.

Osteopathy for endometriosis

Osteopaths are registered allied health practitioners who focus on the bones, muscles, nerves and other tissues that support the human body and control its movements.

How osteopathy can help endometriosis

Osteopathy is a holistic manual therapy focusing on the body's structure and function. For individuals with endometriosis, osteopathy can offer several benefits.

Pain relief

Osteopaths use hands-on techniques to relieve muscle tension, improve blood flow and reduce inflammation, which can help alleviate the chronic pelvic pain associated with endometriosis. Techniques such as myofascial release, gentle mobilisations and soft tissue massage can target body areas often affected by the pain and tension related to endometriosis.

Improved circulation and lymphatic drainage

Osteopathic treatments can help improve circulation, which may reduce the buildup of scar tissue and adhesions that can occur with endometriosis. Better circulation also supports the immune system and helps remove waste products from the body, potentially reducing inflammation.

Pelvic health

Osteopaths often focus on the alignment and function of the pelvis and surrounding structures. By addressing imbalances or restrictions in the pelvis, osteopathy can help alleviate pelvic pain, improve mobility and enhance overall pelvic health.

Stress reduction

Chronic pain from endometriosis can lead to increased stress and tension, which may exacerbate symptoms. Osteopathy can help by promoting relaxation and reducing stress through gentle, calming techniques, which can positively impact overall wellbeing.

Holistic approach

Osteopaths consider the whole body in their treatment plans, considering factors like posture, lifestyle and emotional health. This comprehensive approach can help address not just the physical symptoms of endometriosis but also the associated emotional and psychological challenges.

Dr Lisa Gadd on different endo therapies

Endo warrior and founder of Living Health Group in Melbourne, Lisa has a masters in Osteopathy, a science degree and over 15+ years experience working in the health and fitness industry. Over the years she has worked with many AFL clubs and trains athletes.

Lisa helps explain different therapies and how they support those with endometriosis.

Cupping

This therapy is based on the principle that suction from the cups draws the skin up and mobilises blood and energy around the body, encouraging the body's natural healing process. It can help reduce pain, inflammation and muscle tightness, improve blood flow (circulation), and increase your body's mobility and flexibility. It leaves red marks on your skin for up to a week.

Dry needling

Dry needling is a technique where thin needles are inserted into specific muscle points, known as trigger points, to relieve pain and tension. It can be beneficial for managing the musculoskeletal pain associated with endometriosis.

Targeted muscle pain relief

Endometriosis often causes referred pain, where the pain experienced in one area of the body is actually due to issues in another, such as the lower back, hips or abdomen. Dry needling can target and release tight muscles and trigger points contributing to this pain, providing relief.

Reduction of muscle tension

The chronic pain and inflammation caused by endometriosis can lead to muscle tightness and spasms. Dry needling helps to relax these muscles, improving flexibility and reducing discomfort.

Enhanced blood flow and healing

Dry needling stimulates the targeted muscles, improving blood flow to the area, promoting healing and reducing inflammation. This can help manage pain and improve the function of the affected muscles.

Neuromuscular reset

Dry needling can help reset how nerves communicate with muscles, reducing the pain signals sent to the brain and decreasing pain levels.

Benefits of massage for endometriosis

Multiple studies indicate that regular massage therapy can provide both short-term and long-term relief from pelvic pain and muscle spasms associated with endometriosis. Research has shown that massage can effectively reduce painful menstruation caused by endometriosis. Techniques such as myofascial release can specifically address tight connective tissues, enhancing flexibility and reducing pain.

Lisa says, 'Massage therapy can offer a variety of benefits for individuals who have endometriosis'. Here are ten ways massage may help in managing endometriosis.

1. *Pain relief: Massage therapy can help alleviate the chronic pelvic pain associated with endometriosis by relaxing tense muscles and reducing the pressure on painful areas.*
2. *Improved circulation: Massage promotes better blood circulation, which can help reduce inflammation and improve the healing of tissues affected by endometriosis.*
3. *Stress reduction: Endometriosis often causes stress due to chronic pain and discomfort. Massage helps activate*

the parasympathetic nervous system, which lowers stress hormones and promotes relaxation.

4. *Reduction of muscle tension: Massage helps release muscle tension and spasms common in individuals with endometriosis, particularly in the lower back, abdomen and pelvic area.*
5. *Enhanced lymphatic drainage: Certain massage techniques can stimulate the lymphatic system, helping to reduce swelling and flush out toxins, which may alleviate some symptoms of endometriosis.*
6. *Improved mobility and flexibility: Regular massage can help loosen tight muscles and connective tissue, improving overall mobility and flexibility, especially in the pelvic region.*
7. *Better sleep: Massage can induce relaxation, which can lead to improved sleep quality. Endometriosis pain and discomfort often disrupt sleep.*
8. *Emotional support: The nurturing touch of massage can provide emotional comfort and support, helping individuals feel more cared for and reducing feelings of anxiety or depression related to their condition.*
9. *Hormonal balance: Some types of massage can help balance hormones by stimulating the endocrine system: serotonin (impacting irritability, depression, pain and behaviour), dopamine (impacting intuition, inspiration, joy, enthusiasm, focus and attention span) and epinephrine (impacting reactions to short-term and long-term stress, fatigue and drowsiness), which might help manage the hormonal imbalances that can exacerbate endometriosis symptoms.*
10. *Adhesion management: Gentle massage techniques can help break down adhesions caused by endometriosis, improving tissue mobility and reducing pain associated with these adhesions.*

Be aware

Be careful choosing an allied health practitioner, make sure they are registered. It is essential to work with a qualified massage therapist who understands endometriosis and can tailor the treatment to your specific needs. Regular sessions may help manage symptoms over time, improving quality of life.

Be prepared

If you have private health insurance, check to see if osteopathy is covered. Some health funds have preferred providers who charge less for members.

Psychological support

Cognitive behavioural therapy and acceptance and commitment therapy are commonly used by mental health professionals to help women+ with persistent pelvic pain. These therapies can help patients understand the link between thoughts, emotions and pain, and develop coping strategies.

Learning about chronic pain mechanisms and how pain affects the body and mind can help better manage symptoms. Understanding the nature of persistent pelvic pain empowers those living with it to take control and try different strategies to reduce their pain.

Physical activity and exercise

Staying active is crucial, even though many women+ with pelvic pain may avoid movement due to fear of exacerbating pain. Low-impact activities like swimming or walking can help reduce pain sensitivity. It is recommended that you work with a multidisciplinary healthcare team to develop a tailored physical activity plan.

Mind-body practices

Yoga, stretching (see page 176) and relaxation exercises can help manage pelvic pain. These practices can reduce tension in the pelvic floor, abdominal and hip muscles, which often become tight in response to chronic pain.

Pacing activities

Learning to pace physical activities is important to avoid pain flares while gradually increasing activity levels. This involves finding a balance between doing enough to improve pain without causing exacerbation. We'll cover Spoon Theory in Chapter 12.

Stress management

Stress can amplify pain sensations, so it's crucial to learn to reduce and manage stress. Techniques such as deep breathing, meditation and guided imagery can be helpful.

Sleep hygiene

Improving sleep quality is essential for managing chronic pain. Establishing a consistent sleep schedule, creating a comfortable sleep environment, and practising relaxation techniques before bed can be beneficial.

Emotional support

Seeking support from friends, family or support groups can help combat feelings of isolation and provide emotional relief. Open communication with partners about the impact of pain on relationships and sexual function is also important.

Women with endometriosis often experience a range of emotional challenges, including depression, anxiety and feelings of isolation. This emotional burden can extend to their partners, who may feel helpless, frustrated or worried about their loved one's health. Studies indicate that male partners frequently report experiencing similar emotional distress, including feelings of sadness and anxiety related to their partner's condition.

Effective communication can become strained as partners navigate the complexities of managing a chronic illness. Differences in how each partner perceives and copes with the condition can lead to misunderstandings and conflict. For instance, one partner may view endometriosis as a manageable condition, while the other may see it as a significant obstacle to their future family planning. This mismatch can create tension and feelings of disconnect within the relationship.

Couples facing the challenges of endometriosis may benefit from counselling or therapy to improve communication, enhance emotional support and address intimacy issues. Professional guidance can help couples develop coping strategies and foster a deeper understanding of each other's experiences.

Reflecting on her endo challenges: Patty's story

Patty Pardillo is an endo warrior who describes endometriosis as a 'very temperamental, evil and aggressive beast'. Coming from a non-English-speaking background, her journey was compounded when she needed surgery at 16 years of age. It was 1992 and we knew so much less about endometriosis then, although sadly, not much has changed in terms of treatment.

Patty has lived through seven surgeries since she was 16, including adhesion removal, Mirena insertion, hysterectomy and bowel resection, plus investigative surgeries in between.

She and Joseph were high school sweethearts who went on to get married and have three wonderful children. Joseph calls himself an 'endo sherpa', signifying his commitment to helping Patty carry the load. Things were great until Patty turned 40, and her endometriosis went from dormant to on fire. Patty is now in a good place again with her endometriosis, but it's come with a huge toll, both personally and within their relationship.

She would give her 16-year-old self this advice:

Seek specialist support and advice from the start, and don't just settle for any initial consultation—see the best in the field and leave no stone unturned, as one wrong diagnosis or surgery can actually make it 100 times worse off.

To help manage symptoms, Patty says, 'At the time of its peak and most painful moments, just focusing on family and prayer…combined with meditation and breathing techniques helps me.'

As a mother of three with two daughters, she is concerned about genetic links and says she hopes the next five years will bring:

…effective solutions to remedy the pain and suffering of many others like me, but most importantly, that we learn what causes this bad disease and how we can ultimately prevent it—I hope that there is also more training in the professional field to really get on top of it as well as more investment/research overall.

If either of her daughters started showing symptoms, she would 'Make an appointment with an endo specialist without delay—particularly an excision specialist. Book an appointment to have a detailed endometriosis ultrasound (DIE) scan'. Patty says she would 'Leave no stone unturned and not take shortcuts with this hideous disease!'

First and foremost—It's not okay and normal for you to suck it up and experience excruciating pain and heavy bleeding during and in between your periods!

You are reading this because this disease is real and requires proper planning and detailed attention. That's the first piece of advice that I'd like to underline…

Surround yourself with fellow endo warriors. One of the hidden blessings of my journey was meeting, being inspired by and drawing strength from fellow sufferers, carers and genuine people who truly care about understanding and beating this disease. Don't be a superhero and quietly try navigating through it alone because you think you may just be overreacting or being a drama queen. You're not.

Don't band-aid the solution because endometriosis is a very temperamental, evil and aggressive beast. See an excision specialist and treat with caution other alternatives, such as ablation.

I'm certainly no medical professional by any means, but 'barbecuing' my uterus and adhesions and just burning the surface of my endometriosis turned my condition and symptoms into a raging and angry inferno!

Seek the best-of-the-best advice and don't settle for anything less unless you want to go down the path of a roller-coaster ride of surgeries, ambulance trips and pain-killer cocktails.

Hold on tight to your best friend in between... The best friend I refer to is the hot water bottle!

What you are feeling is real and not just in your head. It's not normal, and you, therefore, need the proper attention and care to plan your journey meticulously.

Connect yourself with a community and network of fellow endo warriors — because knowledge is fundamental and you don't want to rush yourself into any quick fix. Endometriosis is complex and needs specialist attention. Stay the course, have faith and believe.

Integrative health

Integrative health employs multimodal interventions, which may include:
- conventional health care: medications, physical rehabilitation and psychotherapy
- complementary approaches: acupuncture, yoga, herbal medicine and nutritional therapy.

It aims to treat the whole person, not just a health problem. It uses an evidence-based approach to improve health and wellness.

In essence, integrative health is about maintaining a balanced state of wellbeing across all dimensions. Unfortunately, for those with pelvic pain, suspected or diagnosed endometriosis, the journey is one of rejection, judgement, missed diagnoses and delays in treatment.

The relationship between patients and healthcare providers is important. Patients are equal partners in the health management process. A respectful patient-provider relationship and coordination among providers are fundamental.

Body image

Those living with endometriosis describe feeling 'less', no longer a whole person and damaged in some way. Many will talk about their body betraying them or turning against them. It always sounds like a war has started within their body and that they battle with the enemy within. The psychological impact of this attitude is fundamentally unhelpful as hating your own body or part of your own body has the potential to lead to more significant psychological issues, such as body dysmorphic disorder (excessive worry about appearance) and, more commonly, anxiety and depression. The challenge is to learn to accept what we find challenging and reflect on all the hard work our bodies do to help us.

Endometriosis significantly negatively impacts the perception of body image. Prioritising body acceptance, self-compassion and seeking support from healthcare professionals knowledgeable about endometriosis and body image can help.

Research shows that those with endometriosis, which can cause visible changes like scarring from surgery, weight gain from hormonal therapy, and paleness from heavy bleeding and anaemia, have a poorer body image compared to those without the condition. These appearance-based changes contribute to body image distress.

Endometriosis can lead to functional and physical limitations and impaired sexual, reproductive and overall health. The inability to engage in activities due to pain or other symptoms negatively impacts confidence, and everyday challenges like pain, bloating and digestive issues can significantly impact how you perceive and relate to your body.

You need powerful tools to cope with endometriosis and other chronic illnesses. Improving self-esteem and emotional coping strategies can contribute to better psychological outcomes.

Be aware

Body image concerns in endometriosis has been linked to higher rates of depression and anxiety, and low self-esteem. Negative body image can lead to feelings of low self-worth, which, in turn, increases depressive symptoms over time. Visit Body Image Movement www.bodyimagemovement.com.

Your GP can provide a mental health treatment plan, which makes you eligible for ten individual and ten group sessions with a mental health professional each calendar year.

Be prepared

Strategies will help on those bad days, and Health Direct suggests some of the following techniques:

- Focus on your positive qualities, skills and talents.
- Try positive self-talk and avoid negative self-talk.
- Appreciate what your body can do.
- Look at the different body shapes of the people you like and love.
- Set health goals rather than weight-related goals.
- Don't compare your body shape to other people's.
- Unfollow people on social media whose posts trigger negative body image thoughts.
- Visit Butterfly Foundation for support (butterfly.org.au/).

Navigating body image: Sophie's story

Sophie Dillman is a well-loved actress most familiar to Aussies as Ziggy Astoni from Summer Bay. She was on *Home and Away* from 2017 until 2023, and during that time, her character had a drama-filled life being kidnapped, getting married, divorced and having a baby.

Multidisciplinary care **133**

Sophie has also experienced challenges in her real life, being diagnosed with endometriosis at age 21.

I started having symptoms from essentially when I first got my period, but I didn't think a lot of it until I got out of school. I was doing a lot of professional or high-level sports at the time, and I wasn't menstruating much. When I returned to having regular periods, I was throwing up and fainting. The bleeding was heavy, I was really tired and I would be in lectures at university and fall asleep all the time.

She thinks many women+ ignore period symptoms and 'get on with it. She says, 'When I was doing my nursing training, I don't remember having any mention of women+'s health at all, and that's sad.'

At uni, because of the pain, I stretched all the time, and I made sure that I was moving, but it didn't make sense. I was having aches and pains. I could never wear jeans to uni because, by the end of the day, I'd have to have my buttons undone because I'd be so swollen. I just put that down to me, you know, potentially having a poor diet or thinking really bad things about my body. In hindsight, after being diagnosed, it all makes sense as to why those things were occurring, and I was probably really, really harsh on myself. It affected my body image.

Sophie has had three laparoscopic surgeries so far, and was told by the doctor:

You've got endometriosis. We can't do much about it. You're probably going to find it challenging to have a baby, so you should think about doing that sooner rather than later—that was the only guidance I was given. It was only through my research I learnt more.

As a 21-year-old, who's just started my acting degree, I was still a baby myself. I had no idea who I was or what I wanted or anything like that. To have a doctor say, time's ticking, you've got to get on it, because probably, it's the only way that you're to have a baby, and it'll probably help and cure your endometriosis. It was also wrong; it's just such poor practice.

She said it was a complicated scenario when the writers of *Home and Away* came to her with a pregnancy storyline and said:

'Look, this is what we're thinking, but we understand your health journey, and we don't want to put you in a position that makes you upset or gives you any anxiety or anything. So if this is not something you're comfortable with, we won't do it.'

There were occasions when I was playing pregnant that I wouldn't have to wear the bump', she shares. Being pregnant on the show 'was fun to do in a hypothetical sense, especially with my real-life partner [fellow actor Patrick O'Connor]. We fought over names, who changed the first nappy, and everything else.'

Sophie's endo symptoms are often challenging for the wardrobe department, too.

My swelling, of course, comes when I'm stressed. I would be stressing about whether I will fit into my costume that day, every day. I had a really understanding, beautiful wardrobe department that was so kind. When the bloating happened, when the dress wouldn't do up, we had all these little tips and tricks of how I would sit if I needed to keep something undone or have my pants undone until I was rolling up and then do them up.

If there were days that I couldn't wear a bikini or I was really bloated, I tried not to think of the bloating. It is very hard, to be honest, to do a show that is focused on the beach and all those beautiful bodies and everything. But I tried not to think about my bloating from the perspective that it made me look bad.

However, when I had my period, I'd constantly be checking or asking someone to check for blood stains if I was wearing a light colour or if I really like a light fabric or something. It would surely be awkward to have those photos in the media of 'Sophie's period leaking on set.'

As an actor, frolicking on the beach in bikinis and stressing about fitting into costumes affected her body image. She says she was grateful for the 'good grace of my workplace'.

I couldn't hide the endometriosis. You could see it. I walked around with a water bottle most days, and everyone knew I had to carry it. I was very open in the conversations that I had with people about the fact that I had endometriosis, and this is my daily reality. I will have to sit down at certain times and often use a hot water bottle.

Everyone was really understanding. I had directors where I'd tell them, 'Look, I'm really sorry. I'm really swollen today. That's not going to be a flattering shot.' I had a couple of endo surgeries during my stint on the show, and they were so understanding. They gave me all the time off that I needed.

The most important thing that I made sure of was that I wasn't shy about that conversation, where you explain what endometriosis is, and maybe someone will get uncomfortable hearing that for the first time, but afterwards, it's not a problem. Everyone could have handed me my hot water bottle. Everyone could have handed me a pad. You know, it was normalised.

She uses exercise to manage symptoms:

Exercise is a very fine line because they say that high-intensity interval training is great for pain relief, but that can also bring on a flare.

I stretch at least once, probably twice a day, and do some yoga. However, if you overstretch, that can cause a flare-up. Doing yoga means you have to turn on the pelvic floor and hold that really strong, and sometimes that can cause a flare-up. So I find that I just think the key is I have lots of different outlets to use, and if one isn't working at the time, I have to flip to the other one. I try really hard not to feel bad about that. If I can't do a really big session that day or a session that day, I try not to beat myself up too much; I need to accept what I can and can't do every day.

Sophie uses 'hot and cold therapies, hot and cold plunges, and I do think that that helps with my swelling'.

> *I have done acupuncture if I'm having a bad run of pain. I do a lot of dry needling as well. A lot of my pain ends up in my hips.*
>
> *The biggest thing for me is reducing any inflammatory foods. Moving to the UK was a big adjustment because the diet is very different. It is really hard to get a lot of really good-quality produce or gluten-free products.*
>
> *The moment I have something too inflammatory, I'm out for the count for a while now. I avoid any soft dairy, so I don't have cow's milk.*

Sophie knows the chances are that she'll be challenged with fertility, 'but having a baby isn't on my path right now'.

> *The story on* Home and Away *prompted conversations ... I have had many anxious moments and conversations with people about the fact that if I carry a baby, I have to give up my body, which is what I use for my work, and it may not ever look the same or work the same. Then afterwards, I have a child that I'll be feeding. It's different for male actors because they don't have the physical evidence of a baby that changes their path.*
>
> *I definitely think about that a lot. My partner and I both want to have children, but we also don't want to do it when we're not ready ... My mum had a hysterectomy in her 40s. It has crossed my mind about passing endometriosis down; it does really worry me. My hope is that there is potentially some development in research to manage it better and, ultimately, find a cure.*

Bloating and fears about heavy bleeding often cause Sophie stress as an actor, but also in her personal life.

> *My little sister got married earlier this year and four months out, she messaged me and said, 'My period's coming on my wedding day. This is going to be horrendous.' So we started going through questions about the dress doing up. You need to have a checklist for*

endo, the uninvited guest. Wedding days and other precious events are meant to be memories of love and a beautiful moment; instead, they are riddled with fear and anxiety and what-ifs. When I get married, I often think I will have to have one with elastic if I wear a white dress. I can bloat as much as possible and be comfortable because otherwise, I'm just going to panic the whole day.

Sophie believes school education for girls and boys needs to be funded. It needs to go to mums as well, through their daughters, from their GP and their community.

The biggest message is that periods aren't meant to be debilitating. You're not meant to miss life because of your period. And if you are, there should be investigations done. Women aren't meant to live in pain or fear of pain. Whereas it feels like a lot of us do and just suck it up because this is what, you know, the cross that we were given. That's just not the case. If men had endometriosis, it'd be cured by now. If men had periods, they'd get that time off every month. We need to do better.

CHAPTER 10

Relationships

Watching your child in pain is one of the most heart-wrenching experiences a parent can endure. It's a feeling of profound helplessness and an intense desire to alleviate their suffering. The sight of your child in distress grips your heart, creating an emotional ache that mirrors their physical or emotional discomfort.

Seeing my daughter Brianna in pain from the age of eight, her small, trembling body, the way she'd cling to me for comfort, looking at me with a plea, 'Mummy, make it stop', or her attempts to hide her pain to appear brave are overwhelming, even today. As a mature woman and mother herself, I still feel compelled to take her pain away, into myself to spare her any suffering.

In these moments, I oscillate between various emotions — anger at the situation causing the pain (endo and adeno), frustration at my inability to 'fix it', and overwhelming love that drives me to do everything within my power to provide comfort and support to her and others living with endo. That has motivated me to be an advocate and write this book.

I first learnt about endometriosis when I was pregnant with Brianna through the late and great Professor David Healy, whom I mention in the dedication and the acknowledgements of the book. I remember him visiting my MP electorate office. I was hoping I wouldn't throw up because of morning (all-day) sickness, and I also recall being nervous about pronouncing endo... meeee... what now?

Advocating for your child: Brianna's mum's story

Brianna started experiencing what I told her were 'stitches' while playing netball in her first season in under 10s. She also complained when she was riding her bike, especially up hills, and I'd tell her to use her 'pink power' to keep going.

When she started complaining about 'tummy pain' and 'poo getting stuck', we put it down to food intolerances to dairy and wheat. I regret to say my mum and I also put her complaints down to the disruption of her little sister's birth when Brianna was seven.

She started to become doubled over in pain, her face contorted and fists white from clenching. Usually, she would take herself to the toilet, thinking the severe cramps were related to needing to poo. Then, while experiencing excruciating pain, she started bleeding from the vagina. I was in shock and very concerned about what could cause this at her age.

I took her to the local hospital emergency department and was told it was probably appendicitis. I'd had mine out aged 16 and remembered the pain hitting me like a freight train. It did not explain the bleeding. The attending doctor and nurses had no explanation for that. They did query sexual assault, as required under the Victorian mandatory reporting laws.

Brianna's pain continued, and we attended the health care merry-go-round all endo warriors are familiar with: GPs, ultrasound and finally, gynaecologists, and I am grateful to her treating specialists Tony, Jim and Mei. Suspecting endometriosis early on did not vary the treatment for Brianna; transvaginal ultrasound didn't pick up endo as well as it does today, and the only definitive diagnosis was laparoscopic surgery, which we wanted to avoid until absolutely necessary.

Her bleeding became a regular menstrual cycle, accompanied by spotting most weeks. She started on the 'pill', and I remember her being so embarrassed at school when going on camps because medication needed to be handed to the teacher. Concerns about her reputation, presumptions of sexual activity and needing contraception continue to plague girls.

Despite the bleeding and the pain, Brianna was a passionate swimmer, competing in 10-kilometre endurance and 24-hour relay swim meets. She also played water polo in the firsts at school and worked as a swimming teacher. She played netball, AFL football and remains fit through Pilates, Kayla's Sweat app and weights.

Endo has invaded her life in ways familiar to endo warriors; wearing white for her school formal and the wedding was stressful; she had a cyst burst Christmas night a couple of years ago, and she has endured excruciating pain, so visible on her face, during sporting finals, the day of her grade 8 piano exam and VCE finals.

Brianna always wanted to be an architect and started in her university course of choice before deciding to switch to nursing. Her first job out of uni was in the busy Monash Health emergency department, and she started there in March 2020, remaining through the COVID-19 pandemic. Navigating endo pain in a frantic environment wearing plastic personal protective equipment (PPE) was challenging.

She is now a fertility nurse, again motivated by her endo and adeno journey, following the birth of my grandson Oliver in August 2022.

She and her 'high school sweetheart' husband, Daniel, a paramedic, have endured the challenges of navigating their relationship through the tumultuous storm that is this insidious disease. I am so incredibly proud of the resilient, strong, motivated ball of energy she is. I wish every day I could take her pain away.

Her most recent laparoscopic surgery, while I was writing this book, removed endo from her bowel, rectum and ovary, and they finally removed her appendix, which was blamed for her pain 20 years before.

Dads as endo supporters

From a gender equity perspective, involving men in their daughters' lives, their wives' lives, and their sisters' lives, educating them about this terrible disease called endometriosis and the consequences for a woman+, is lacking. It's difficult enough and challenging enough to have girls and women+ understand that painful periods are not normal.

Ellie Angel-Mobbs says:

I don't think there is anything more harrowing for a dad than to see his daughter in pain and be powerless to stop it.

I want to acknowledge my dad who is just the most incredible father to me and husband to Mum during such a harrowing time in her life. A lot of men wouldn't know how to deal with that, especially decades ago. He's really such a Mendo champion. He's done so much work being the male voice for endometriosis in our family and community.

We need to support men, too. I know here, in my workplace, they've just introduced that they're allowing men to have extended paternity leave. And they can also get carers' leave too, if their partner needs it. It's once again around creating that awareness and... once places start doing it, then other people will get on board, and hopefully, we'll see this change over the future. The men in our lives and those partners in our lives are just so important.

My message is: if your man isn't supporting you with endo it's a big red flag. Flick them off; you can do so much better.

Endometriosis and its impact on intimate relationships

Endometriosis can profoundly affect intimate relationships, influencing both partners emotionally and physically. Recognising these effects is essential for maintaining a healthy relationship.

Women with endometriosis often experience dyspareunia (painful intercourse), leading to the avoidance of sexual activity. This not only impacts physical intimacy but can also create emotional distance as partners deal with the pain and discomfort during sex. This and fatigue associated with endometriosis can lead to feelings of inadequacy or guilt, making individuals feel like a burden to their partners. This emotional toll can cause tension and misunderstandings within the relationship.

Many endo warriors find it challenging to communicate their symptoms and needs effectively. They may fear that discussing painful experiences will upset their partner or lead to feelings of helplessness on both sides. Open communication is crucial for couples dealing with endometriosis. Discussing how the condition affects daily life, including intimacy and emotional wellbeing, fosters understanding and support between partners.

Partners may experience their own emotional struggles, including frustration, helplessness or sadness about their loved one's condition. If not addressed openly, this shared burden can affect the overall relationship dynamic.

It's important for partners to be involved in discussions about treatment options and emotional support. This involvement helps them understand the condition better and allows for shared coping strategies.

Discussing endometriosis should occur in a calm, distraction-free environment where both partners feel comfortable expressing their feelings. Use 'I' statements to express personal experiences without placing blame. For example, saying 'I feel pain during intercourse' instead of 'You make me feel pain' fosters a more supportive dialogue.

Couples can explore other forms of intimacy that do not involve penetration, such as cuddling or gentle touch, to maintain closeness while managing symptoms. Experimenting with different positions or timing sexual activity around less painful times in the menstrual cycle can help find what works best for both partners.

Having the right support: Emma's story

Dr Emma Watkins is Australia's sweetheart. An entertainer for all ages and stages, she was the first female member of The Wiggles from 2013 to 2021.

She is genuine, empathetic and passionate about enhancing the lives of her audience and fellow endo warriors. In late August, we appeared on Channel 7's *The House of Wellness*, interviewed by my friend Jo Stanley, and I was an emotional mess when I arrived. Brianna was in critical care in the hospital after a challenging birth, while my grandson Oliver was in neonatal intensive care in the Royal Children's Hospital in Melbourne. Even though I misspoke some figures, Emma soothed me enough to be coherent when speaking about endometriosis and adenomyosis.

After years of frequent heavy periods, pain and exhaustion leading to her collapsing on several occasions while on tour, Emma finally sought a 'name for her pain'. She was diagnosed with stage 4 endometriosis in April 2017 by gynaecologist Professor Jason Abbott.

This diagnosis led to recognition of the impact endometriosis was having on her life and marked a pivotal change in her career. Emma moved away from the rigorous touring schedule that characterised her time with The Wiggles, which often involved performing extensively throughout the year. She retired from her role as the much-loved Yellow Wiggle in 2021 to focus on her health journey.

Her status as an endo warrior has led her to prioritise her health and wellbeing, pursuing projects that align with her physical capabilities while continuing to engage in creative and advocacy efforts that resonate with her personal experiences and values. She has completed a PhD and through her character, Emma Memma, she uses visual language, movement and dance to offer more communication options for children and their family networks. Emma tells her story:

I experienced terrible period pain in high school. I was really unwell, and it got to the point I was bleeding every day. I didn't realise I had endometriosis; I didn't really know what the symptoms were.

While touring around the world with The Wiggles, I didn't understand that the pain I suffered wasn't normal; as a result, I didn't seek medical care for way too long. I was a bit lazy and, in retrospect, I was about ten years late, which no doubt contributed to the development of chocolate cysts.

Since I was diagnosed, worrying about the future, the impact of the disease on my life, and potential motherhood and future fertility has weighed heavily.

After having laparoscopic surgery, I felt better in the following months, but it took years to rehabilitate my body and get on top of managing my symptoms. Speculation about my cancellations

144 The Australian Guide to Living Well with Endometriosis

for booked performances being due to pregnancy was confronting, especially when I was only just learning about the statistics on fertility challenges. I was deliberately upfront about my endometriosis and recovery from the procedure.

Endometriosis has a way of hovering in my consciousness. Oliver Brian and I married in 2022, and he has been a source of emotional stability for me, especially as I navigate the uncertainties surrounding the challenges of conceiving due to endometriosis. I am so grateful to have a supportive partner who understands the complexities involved. Oliver provides both emotional reassurance and practical assistance and has enabled me to navigate the challenges of endometriosis while pursuing my studies and passions and maintaining a healthy lifestyle to help manage symptoms, and avoid flare-ups and complications.

By sharing my personal endometriosis journey, I aim to reduce stigma and encourage women to seek help when they experience symptoms. I hope to foster a sense of solidarity among women facing the challenges of this invasive disease and help them learn to live well with endometriosis.

Educational resources

Providing partners with reliable information about endometriosis can help them better understand the condition, leading to increased empathy and support.

EndoZone (endozone.com.au) has advice for partners and physical intimacy, and endometriosis on their website (more information is in the resources section). Pelvic Pain Foundation of Australia (pelvicpain .org.au) also has information on the website for women+ experiencing painful sex. You'll find these and more in the resources section.

Couples counselling

Engaging in therapy with a professional experienced in chronic conditions can provide tools for better communication and coping strategies. This can be particularly beneficial if one partner struggles to cope with the emotional aspects of endometriosis.

Endometriosis presents unique challenges to relationships, affecting intimacy and emotional wellbeing. However, through open communication, mutual support and professional guidance, couples can navigate these challenges together. Understanding that both partners are affected by the condition fosters a supportive environment that strengthens their bond while managing the complexities of endometriosis.

With appropriate support and coping strategies, couples can navigate these challenges and maintain fulfilling relationships despite the difficulties posed by endometriosis.

Endometriosis and its impact on family planning

Discussing having a family of your own can be difficult for you and your partner; you may not be on the same timeline, particularly if you have endometriosis, adenomyosis or PCOS and know it may not be as easy as tracking ovulation and having sex.

Deciding to try for a baby is also an emotional roller-coaster, with performance anxiety killing the mood and the weight of expectation when your period is due. When your period arrives, it can prompt a grief response and make you feel like you've failed.

It is common for couples to share feelings of anxiety, fear, sadness, worthlessness and resentment and lash out with blame. All of these emotions can make any existing relationship issues worse. Counselling before starting the pregnancy journey can help air issues, fears and concerns, and manage unhelpful responses and difficult behaviours.

Fertility clinics offer counselling to confront any issues; let you know what to expect, emotionally as well as hormonally; and support you when a cycle doesn't result in eggs, embryos aren't viable or transfers don't result in pregnancy.

For a partner of a woman+ with endometriosis and adenomyosis, it can be like a ménage à trois, a third entity in your relationship. Many of the contributors to this book have spoken about the commitment of their partner, for some their only and lifelong partner, who have taken the 'for better and for worse' literally, be that through sexual challenges, life limitations or fertility challenges.

146 The Australian Guide to Living Well with Endometriosis

Sex and intimacy

Sex and relationship counsellors can help couples with sexual intimacy, pleasure making and lifting libido. They support each person to find pleasure and arousal, involving the whole body, not just 'below the belt'. Sometimes genital touch can trigger the woman+'s pain or even bring on a stress response, which tightens up just when you want to loosen.

Endometriosis commonly causes painful intercourse, which can severely impact sexual intimacy. Partners may experience a loss of desire or fear of causing pain, leading to avoidance of sexual activity altogether. This situation can foster guilt, sadness and frustration for both partners, as they may feel a loss of closeness and affection.

One way to open communication about intimacy is through 'sync set' (itsnormal.com), a deck of cards with conversation starters about desires and challenges developed by certified sex and relationship practitioner Georgia Grace. There are sex toys to explore to excite the clitoris with external vibrators to arouse rather than douse. The OHNUT is one option available through the Pelvic Pain Foundation of Australia, and sales support its important work. It consists of four intimate wearable rings that compress down to act as a soft buffer during sex. These rings allow you to make simple adjustments so you and your partner can discover comfort and what depths feel good—for both of you.

Intimacy beyond sexuality

The impact of endometriosis on intimacy extends beyond sexual relations. Partners may find it challenging to maintain emotional closeness due to the physical and emotional toll of the condition. The stress of managing symptoms, treatment decisions and the uncertainty of the future can lead to social withdrawal and decreased quality time spent together.

Daily life and responsibilities

Endometriosis can significantly affect daily life, including work, household responsibilities and social activities. The individual with the condition may struggle with fatigue and pain, necessitating increased support from their partner. If one partner feels overwhelmed by additional responsibilities, this shift can lead to feelings of resentment or imbalance in the relationship.

Social isolation

Couples may also experience social isolation as they navigate the challenges of endometriosis. Friends and family may not fully understand the condition, leading to a lack of support or companionship. This isolation can exacerbate feelings of loneliness and stress for both partners, further straining the relationship.

Support networks

Building a support network, including friends, family and support groups specifically for couples dealing with endometriosis, can provide valuable emotional relief and practical advice. Sharing experiences with others who understand the challenges can help mitigate feelings of isolation and provide a sense of community.

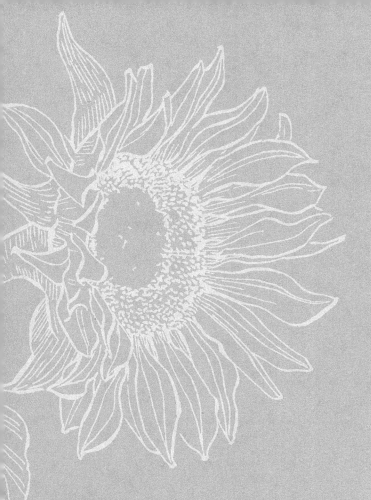

PART IV
Try it out
Holistic lifestyle and self-care

CHAPTER 11

Lifestyle and self-care

According to the World Health Organization, self-care is the ability of individuals, families and communities to manage, promote and maintain their own health and cope with illness with or without the support of a health or care worker.

Chronic pain and other endo symptoms that impact your life can't be managed day to day by doctors and nurses or medication alone. Empowering yourself to manage endometriosis without surgery or pharmaceuticals involves a variety of lifestyle, dietary and alternative therapy approaches.

Over 75 per cent of individuals with endometriosis rely on self-management strategies to cope with their symptoms. These strategies encompass a range of approaches to alleviate pain and improve quality of life. One Australian study found that as many as 89 per cent of women+ with endo manage pain through complementary and self-care in a health system not designed for or flexible enough to include patient-centred, multidisciplinary care.

Endometriosis and adenomyosis do not just affect where lesions grow. It impacts:

- bio: genetics, physical health, and the function of our body and internal organs
- psycho: moods, thinking patterns, and behaviours
- social: culture, family, socioeconomic and relationships, including work.

Put it together—*biopsychosocial*—we need a health system that can support you across all three aspects.

I encourage you to explore evidence-based self-care using proven, reliable and effective methods for promoting overall health, disease prevention and for managing health conditions. These interventions can include:

- medicines: you can use high-quality medications independently or with minimal supervision
- devices: tools or equipment (such as TENS) designed for self-use
- diagnostics: record pain, periods, pee, poo and painful sex
- digital interventions: mobile apps or online platforms to help support you with information and lift you up when you are feeling down.

Self-care encompasses prioritising your physical and mental health and following a treatment plan to support you in managing the symptoms impacting your life. Every day is different, and it is important to have a kit and caboodle with therapies to help you through.

Working with a healthcare team that includes various specialists (e.g. gynaecologists, pain specialists, physiotherapists, psychologists) can provide comprehensive care and address different aspects of chronic pelvic pain.

Integrative medicine can help people with endometriosis symptoms such as pain, fatigue, anxiety, digestive issues, sexual issues and fertility. It's important to note that the treatments promoted in integrative medicine are not substitutes for conventional medical care. They should be used along with standard medical treatment.

'Nothing about us without us'

In the health system context, you are a patient when you are receiving treatment from a health practitioner. The Australian Charter of Health Care Rights states that you have a right to access the healthcare services you need; to receive safe and high-quality health care in a place that makes you feel safe; to be respected as a person along with your culture, identity, beliefs and choices; to work in partnership with health practitioners to make decisions; to receive clear information and access to your own health records; to have your personal privacy respected; and to have the right to share feedback without being worried about consequences for your treatment.

Autonomy for patients means they have the right to decide what is best for them in consideration of their individual context. This includes accepting or declining specific healthcare options, and this further extends to the following to enable patients to make informed decisions through:

- Ethical principles: Informed decision making aligns with the ethical principle that patients should actively participate in their own care. It respects their autonomy and values their preferences.
- Access to relevant information: To make informed decisions, patients need accurate, relevant information. Healthcare providers play a crucial role in providing this information and explaining risks, benefits and alternatives.
- Changing decisions: Patients have the right to change their decisions over time. Flexibility and ongoing communication are essential.

Justice in healthcare means fairness in treatment and access to medical resources. This ensures that all patients receive equitable care regardless of their background or financial situation. It also encompasses the ethical obligation to provide informed consent for all patients, ensuring that marginalised or intersectionally disadvantaged individuals are not treated unfairly. Receiving information in your primary language, for example, is a fundamental right, and patients can request an interpreter service.

Empowering patients with knowledge ensures that healthcare choices are well-informed and aligned with their needs (see Chapter 18 for more on communicating with healthcare providers). All patients should receive care that focuses on the following:

- the whole person: care that treats the individual, not just a health problem; it considers physical, mental, emotional and spiritual needs
- an evidence-based approach: considering the most up-to-date and reliable evidence backed up by research to improve health and wellness

Lifestyle and self-care **153**

- a combination of therapies: using a mix of conventional healthcare approaches (like medication and psychotherapy) with complementary therapies (like acupuncture and yoga).

The relationship between patients and healthcare providers is important. Patients are equal partners in the healing process. Communication among providers aims for well-coordinated care between different providers and specialists.

CHAPTER 12

Diet and nutrition

There is so much conflicting information about diet and what's best for endometriosis. I have long believed that food acts as a preventative and treatment. Personally, I have consulted dietitians and done decades of lay research into what foods can help or hinder my health journey with endometriosis and I have distilled a list of what's recommended for endo in the fridge and cupboard based on research. I recommend you consult a dietitian or nutritionist, and use this as a guide.

Are you what you eat?

According to research, women+ with endometriosis seem to consume fewer vegetables, fruits (particularly citrus fruits), dairy products and foods rich in vitamin D and long-chain omega-3 fatty acids. Long-term studies have shown that a higher intake of citrus fruits is beneficial; women+ consuming more than one serve of citrus a day had a 22 per cent lower risk of endometriosis. They also showed that those eating less than one serve of vegetables in the Brassica genus (e.g. broccoli, cauliflower and kale) had a 13 per cent higher risk of endometriosis.

There is no universal diet that works for all women+ with endometriosis, as the condition is complex and symptoms vary significantly between individuals; however, specific dietary changes may help manage symptoms.

Endometriosis is an inflammatory condition, so, focusing on anti-inflammatory foods, supplements and gut support makes sense to balance that angry endo, to feed the good bacteria and to say good riddance to the bad. A healthy gut microbiome can influence hormone regulation, including estrogen metabolism. This is significant for endometriosis, as estrogen can exacerbate symptoms.

Managing the fuel efficiency of your digestive system is central to overall health and wellbeing. If it is healthy, it takes the pressure off your body so it can focus on fighting endometriosis symptoms, giving you the tools to repair and regrow, and the energy to live well despite the endo. The suggestions in this chapter may not suit everyone, and we are not advocating for particular diets or recommending specific foods.

The types of food listed here are based on research into the good, bad and ugly through academic studies on endometriosis and diet. Good health through a good gut supports a healthy immune system to empower life.

We met Associate Professor Magdalena Simonis AM in Chapter 5, and as a leading women+'s health expert, she prioritises discussions about diet with the women+ who present to her with endo symptoms.

> *If they don't like eating red meat, we need to look at what they're having and what sources of iron they're getting, from what and how often. So for young women who choose a mainly vegetarian diet, I do think that it is well worth taking an iron supplement when they menstruate, restocking the flow you're losing. Then, let's think strategically about how and where you get your iron through your diet throughout the week if you're vegetarian or pescetarian.*

She suggests education about where to source iron, such as legumes, lentils, tofu, eggs, green leafy greens, and other things that provide that.

> *It also depends on the combination of foods and how you have it; for example, if you have a meal and drink coffee immediately after the meal, you might not absorb much iron. You're best keeping caffeine well away from mealtime. Milk and iron don't go well together because they counter the iron absorption and calcium in the milk.*

My mum always said, 'Drink orange juice with your meat', I told my daughters the same. Professor Simonis agrees:

> *Orange juice is the golden standard here. If you don't have orange juice, have a piece of fruit, an apple, a pear. However, if you do have iron deficiency, you need to bump it up. You do need to take a supplement. It's a question of which one, how you take it, and how long you take it for. The more iron deficient you are, the longer you must take it. I say to my patients, if they tend to become constipated, take it every two or three days, it's still better than not taking it at all.*

The daily dozen

I read *How Not to Die* by Dr. Michael Greger and Gene Stone (2015) while looking at how to nourish my health. It has been endorsed by medical experts and some high-profile gurus, including the Dalai Lama and Dan Buettner, author of *The Blue Zones Solution*.

This book changed my life and my diet. Each morning, the Dr. Greger's Daily Dozen app sends me a reminder of the foods I should include in my diet that day. This usually includes the core food, and I have added examples:

- beans (three serves): peanuts (they are actually a legume), one cup of fresh peas, a quarter cup of hummus or bean dip, half a cup of cooked beans (e.g. chickpeas, black beans, cannellini, kidney beans)
- berries (one serve): a quarter cup of dried berries, half a cup of fresh or frozen berries
- other fruits (three serves): avocados, bananas, oranges, cantaloupe, kiwi, oranges, tomatoes
- cruciferous vegetables (one serve): a quarter cup of Brussels or broccoli sprouts, rocket, bok choy, cabbage, cauliflower, kale, watercress, or a tablespoon of horseradish (it is high in sulphur and can cause bloating and gas, but the benefits are worth it)—research shows these vegetables help to lower estrogen levels, as well as regulating blood cholesterol, improving glucose control and being full of fibre, they support bowel health

Diet and nutrition **157**

- greens (two servings): one cup of raw salad leaves, spinach, half a cup of cooked greens
- other vegetables (two serves): potatoes, sweet potato, eggplant, green beans, wombok, carrot, celery, corn, oyster mushroom, olives, spring onion, zucchinis
- flaxseed, aka linseed, one tablespoon ground (avoid the full seed): add to everything—its full of cancer-fighting lignans
- nuts and seeds (one serve; approximately a handful): Brazil nuts, almonds, macadamia, pecan, chia, pumpkin/pepita, sesame, poppy, hemp, pine nuts
- herbs and spices: a quarter of a teaspoon of turmeric in addition to other herbs and spices, such as ginger, saffron, cinnamon, paprika, sage, vanilla, dill, coriander/cilantro and cumin
- whole grains (three serves): sourdough, rice, oats, quinoa, pasta and barley, buckwheat (which isn't wheat), popcorn, rye
- beverages (five serves): water, of course, soda water and especially a good mineral water, which provides magnesium, lowers blood pressure, regulates blood circulation, strengthens bones, promotes digestive health and helps constipation. [I am a tea collector, and love rooibos (lowers blood pressure, improves cholesterol levels and reduces risk of developing cardiovascular disease), chamomile (good for diabetes, menstrual pain and sleep problems), peppermint (helps skin conditions, headaches, cold and flu, nausea and IBS) matcha (antioxidant and anti-inflammatory), jasmine (aroma has a calming effect on the autonomous nervous system and is good for mental clarity and boosting your immune system), dandelion tea (good for reducing inflammation, improving cholesterol levels and urinary tract infections and is a good source of minerals; caution: dandelion can cause an allergic reaction, interfere with medications, and strong tea is high FODMAP).]
- exercise (one serve): 90 minutes of moderate or 40 minutes of vigorous exercise.

Adapting your diet to what works for you

I have followed FODMAP (designed to help people discover which foods are problematic for them; see page 159 for more) for over

20 years, and it immediately improved my digestion and gut health. I personally avoid onion, garlic, apples, dried and stone fruits, processed foods and gluten—although I do eat sourdough as the pre-fermenting process breaks down the 'farty fructans'. I've modified the list to my tastes and tolerances.

I also stopped eating all meat and dairy years ago, but I eat fish. I often have sardines on toast or smoked salmon for breakfast (despite the protests about the smell from the fam) and eggs. I have coffee for my heart function, I don't drink alcohol. Having heaps of protein and iron is important. Many vegan foods are full of wheat, soy and additives, which are worse than whole foods.

This has improved my health by reducing inflammation. I lost the genetic lottery, living with asthma, inflammatory bowel disease, fibromyalgia and postural orthostatic tachycardia syndrome (POTS), and despite my healthy weight and lifestyle, diabetes, like my mum.

If you are trying new foods, please watch for allergic reactions. Always have antihistamines handy, and do not hesitate to call an ambulance.

Low-FODMAP diet

FODMAP stands for 'fermentable oligosaccharides, disaccharides, monosaccharides and polyols'. These are short-chain carbohydrates (sugars) that the small intestine struggles to absorb and that can aggravate a sensitive gut. Research has found that following a restrictive diet and avoiding foods that can trigger digestive symptoms can reduce inflammation and really help those living with endometriosis who suffer from bowel, gut and toileting issues.

Research also suggests that adherence to a low-FODMAP diet may help reduce endometriosis-related pain. In one study, participants who followed this diet reported lower pain scores related to period pain, deep painful sex and chronic pelvic pain after six months compared to their baseline levels.

The low-FODMAP diet encourages individuals to identify specific food triggers that exacerbate their symptoms. This customised approach allows women+ to tailor their diets based on their unique responses to different foods, leading to more effective symptom management.

Ellie Angel-Mobbs has worked out the foods to avoid: 'I watch my diet and have figured out what is best for me with my lymphocytic colitis. I do FODMAP, I avoid red meat, garlic, onion and tomato, which is the biggest no-go zone ever.'

Monash University researchers Dr Peter Gibson and Dr Sue Shepherd discovered FODMAPs in 2005. Dr Shepherd wrote a book, *Low FODMAP Recipes*, with allergen-free, FODMAP-friendly recipes the whole family can enjoy without consequences (there's also an app). The diet essentially comprises a list of foods, and a traffic light system is used to rate foods for fructose, lactose, mannitol, sorbitol, galacto-oligosaccharides (GOS) and fructans (all foods that can aggravate your gut). Trust your gut.

Best low-FODMAP foods for endometriosis

- vegetables: bok choy, bean sprouts, carrots, cucumbers, lettuce, potatoes, spinach, tomatoes, zucchini
- fruits: blueberries, cantaloupe, grapes, kiwi, mandarin oranges, pineapple, raspberries, strawberries
- proteins: eggs, plain cooked meats, poultry, seafood
- grains: gluten-free breads and cereals made from rice, oats, quinoa, corn
- dairy alternatives: lactose-free milk, almond milk, coconut milk, hard cheeses
- nuts and seeds: almonds, macadamia nuts, peanuts, pumpkin seeds, walnuts
- herbs and spices: basil, chives, ginger, lemongrass, olives, parsley, rosemary, thyme.

Worst high-FODMAP foods for endometriosis

- vegetables: artichokes, asparagus, broccoli, Brussels sprouts, cabbage, cauliflower, garlic, onions, mushrooms
- fruits: apples, apricots, blackberries, cherries, figs, mango, nectarines, pears, plums, watermelon, dried fruit
- dairy: milk, yoghurt, soft cheeses, ice cream
- grains: wheat, rye, barley, pasta, breads, cereals
- legumes: beans, lentils, chickpeas
- sweeteners: honey, agave, high fructose corn syrup.

Anti-inflammatory diet

The body uses white blood cells to protect you from injury or infection from outside invaders, such as bacteria and viruses—it directs blood flow to what the brain says is the source. Some chemicals can cause fluid to leak into your tissues, resulting in swelling and other protective processes that can trigger nerves. We have talked about how endometriosis is an inflammatory disease that can impact the entire nervous system.

Chronic inflammation can't be seen, but its impacts are familiar to anyone living with endometriosis and other chronic conditions, such as autoimmune disease, rheumatoid arthritis, asthma, diabetes and inflammatory bowel disease. It can cause abdominal pain, chest pain, fatigue/insomnia, joint pain or stiffness, mouth sores, skin rashes and hormonal acne, depression, anxiety and other mood disorders. Gastrointestinal (GI) issues, like diarrhoea, constipation and acid reflux, are indications of inflammation.

Food can influence inflammation, immune function and hormonal balance. Research shows that incorporating anti-inflammatory foods like omega-3 fatty acids, antioxidants and fibre, minerals and vitamins, as well as superfoods like flaxseeds and seaweed into your diet can be beneficial for managing endometriosis symptoms.

Everyone's digestive system is different, and it is impacted by medications and other conditions you live with. Therefore, it's beneficial to monitor how your body reacts and consult a healthcare professional or registered dietitian for personalised advice. Keeping a food diary to identify personal triggers is helpful.

The following foods should be avoided as they can provoke inflammation:

- red meat
- processed meats like bacon; sausage; smoked, cured, and salted foods; and deli meats like ham are high in inflammatory compounds and should be limited or eliminated
- trans fats and fried food, fast food and processed snacks
- foods with refined carbohydrates, like white bread, pasta and pastries, can spike inflammation
- sugary drinks, lollies, chocolates and desserts
- alcohol can increase estrogen levels and inflammation

- excessive caffeine (more than 300 milligrams per day, about three cups of coffee). Coffee can contain between 100 and 170 milligrams of caffeine per serving, and strong black teas have about 60 milligrams of caffeine. Energy drinks and drinks with guarana can also contain caffeine.

Omega-3 fatty acids

Healthy fats can help manage endometriosis by reducing inflammation, regulating hormones, supporting immune function and alleviating pain. Research has found the anti-inflammatory action of omega-3s helps to alleviate pain and reduce the size of endometriotic lesions, reducing the production of inflammatory prostaglandins that can exacerbate endo symptoms.

Plant-based sources include flaxseeds, chia seeds and walnuts, which provide alpha-linolenic acid (ALA) and omega-3. You can use oils rich in omega-3s, such as flaxseed, rapeseed and canola oil instead of oils high in omega-6 fatty acids (like most vegetable oils, safflower, sunflower, sesame and peanut), which can promote inflammation. Fish oils like cod liver, krill and algae are also great sources.

Fatty fish options rich in omega-3 fatty acids include smoked, canned or fresh trout, salmon, mackerel, sardines (choose olive oil not tomato sauce), tuna, and other sources include oysters, seabass, prawns, seaweed and algae.

Omega-3 supplements, particularly with eicosapentaenoic acid (EPA) and docosahexaenoic acid (DHA), are more effective, and the omega-3s from supplements can vary based on the formulation and individual absorption rates.

To soy or not to soy?

Soy is high in protein, calcium and iron and is available in traditional chalky-looking slabs, marinated packs, soymilk, edamame, soy nuts and sprouts. Fermented soy products include miso, tempeh, nattō and soy sauce. I am a non-dairy eater, and I love tofu sausages and burgers, soy pasta and soymilk yoghurts and cheeses.

The complex relationship between soybeans and endometriosis has generated considerable debate among researchers and healthcare professionals. Science tells us that soybeans are rich in phytoestrogens, particularly isoflavones like genistein and daidzein. These compounds can mimic estrogen in the body, and some studies have found that they 'feed' the endometriosis lesions.

In some studies in which soy was removed from the diet, the participants showed improvements in abnormal bleeding and deceased period pain. Contrary findings from other research have shown no significant difference in phytoestrogen levels between women+ with and without endometriosis, indicating that the relationship is not straightforward.

Whether soy is a friend or foe and might depend on factors such as the form of soy consumed (fermented vs unfermented), the amount and individual responses. So use it in moderation, if at all.

Gut microbiota and endometriosis

Addressing gut health through diet, probiotics and lifestyle changes may offer a complementary approach to traditional treatments for endometriosis, such as hormonal therapies and surgery. This holistic strategy can help improve overall wellbeing and symptom management.

Medical research increasingly recognises the relationship between endometriosis and gut health, highlighting the importance of maintaining a healthy gut microbiome for managing symptoms associated with this condition.

Women+ with endometriosis can have dysbiosis, an imbalance in gut bacteria. This can lead to increased inflammation and immune dysfunction, which can impact the development of endometriosis lesions. The gut microbiome is also involved in the metabolism of estrogen. Dysbiosis can disrupt this process, potentially leading to elevated estrogen levels.

Some studies suggest that women+ with endometriosis may experience increased intestinal permeability, often called 'leaky gut'. This condition allows toxins and bacteria to enter the bloodstream, triggering further inflammation and immune responses that can exacerbate endometriosis.

Gut health and your microbiome

Research indicates that probiotic supplementation may help alleviate symptoms of endometriosis by restoring a healthy gut microbiome, the family of bacteria, yeast and fungi that live in your digestive system.

It is important to know the difference between pre, pro- and postbiotics.

- Probiotics are live micro-organisms that maintain or improve the balance of good to bad bacteria in your digestive system. They can enhance immune function and reduce inflammation, potentially leading to improved pain management and quality of life for those affected by endometriosis.
- Prebiotics act as nutrition for gut bacteria, helping them to flourish. When we eat plant-based fibre, it feeds the good bacteria, which keep our digestive system healthy. If you eat foods that irritate or inflame the digestive system, like FODMAP foods for those who are intolerant, it can be as harmful as a diet high in processed, sugary and fatty foods, because they feed the bad bacteria. This can lead to an unbalanced microbiome.
- Prebiotics are typically high in fructans and oligosaccharides, the 'O' in FODMAP, and include soy, onion, garlic, artichokes and wheat, chickpeas, lentils, barley and oats, all of which should be avoided on the low-FODMAP diet. You are best to take a supplement if these foods bother you.
- Postbiotics are created by the fermentation process and can slow down the growth of bad bacteria.

As well as helping overall gut health, foods high in fibre also help eliminate excess estrogen, reducing its absorption in the colon—you literally poo it out.

Antioxidants and gut health

Antioxidants include zinc and vitamins A, C, and E, which are found in citrus like oranges, mangoes, carrots, sweet potatoes, pumpkin and other orange foods, kiwi fruit, berries, broccoli, spinach, cabbage, kale and tomatoes. Dark chocolate, which is high in cocoa, contains antioxidant flavanols, which can reduce oxidative stress and inflammation, and a number of research studies suggest that they may reduce pelvic pain.

Another compound, cysteine, is an amino acid found in most high-protein foods, like fish, meat, soy, dairy, and grains. It can heal the gut and promote a healthy gut microbiome. When taken as a supplement, it is usually in the form of N-acetyl-L-cysteine (NAC). The body makes this into cysteine and then into glutathione, a powerful antioxidant and anti-inflammatory. It has also been shown to positively impact fertility and egg quality. A recent study found oral NAC reduces endometriosis-related pain and the size of endometriomas.

Benefits of fermented foods

Fermented foods can ensure that essential vitamins and minerals are more readily absorbed and positively mitigate the risk of estrogen-related issues. They are also rich in probiotics.

The consumption of fermented foods can promote the production of short-chain fatty acids (SCFAs), which have anti-inflammatory properties. This is particularly important for endometriosis, as inflammation is a central feature of the condition. SCFAs can help lower inflammation locally in the gut and systemically throughout the body.

They can aid digestion, making managing gastrointestinal discomfort easier for individuals with endometriosis. This is especially beneficial for individuals with endometriosis, as they may have increased nutritional needs due to chronic inflammation.

Some of the best fermented foods to include in the diet are:
- lacto-fermented vegetables: kimchi and sauerkraut are high in lactobacillus strains that support gut health
- kefir and yoghurt: cultured dairy products that are rich in probiotics and can be beneficial, especially for lactose-intolerant people, as the culturing process breaks down lactose
- kombucha: fermented tea containing beneficial bacteria, which can also be a refreshing beverage option (make sure it has no added sugar).

Dr Eliza Colgrave on balancing diet and exercise

I was speaking at a women+'s leadership summit in Canberra when I met Dr Eliza Colgrave over a little food table set aside for 'irritable' people. We bonded over speculation about the dry-looking morsels on offer compared with the abundance of food on the main buffet.

Eliza talked about being a gluten-free coeliac on a plant-based diet to manage her endometriosis, and the penny dropped—we'd heard of each other in the endo community. Eliza is a highly respected early career researcher I had heard about from gurus Professor Peter Rogers and Associate Professor Sarah Holdsworth-Carson from the University of Melbourne.

Eliza is committed to finding answers about the insidious condition that has caused her pelvic pain and cramping, heavy menstrual bleeding, brain fog, fatigue and digestive issues since she was 11 years old. She remembers she 'always pushed through the pain at school and would spend some classes in the bathroom during real bad flare-ups'.

Finally, her mum convinced her that the pain wasn't normal. She was diagnosed with endometriosis at age 18: 'I feel like we've done a really good job over the last decade raising awareness, but at the time, I hadn't heard about it in school and Mum hadn't even heard of it, so it was a bit terrifying as well.'

Eliza is grateful to her gynaecologist, who was 'very clued into the fact that maybe it was worth seeing a gastroenterologist'. Sure enough, she was eventually diagnosed with coeliac disease, an autoimmune disease that causes an intolerance to gluten in the small intestine, and can cause similar symptoms to endometriosis. 'Having both endometriosis and coeliac treated really improved my quality of life. Obviously, it's all happening in your pelvis and can aggravate each other.'

After her second laparoscopic surgery, she learnt she had suspected adenomyosis:

My specialist said, if she didn't know me, she would have said, by looking at my uterus, I was a 40-year-old woman postpartum, post having children. Instead, I was an 18-year-old girl working out what the hell was going on with her body. Like so many people, I'm carrying that wonderful trifecta [endometriosis, adenomyosis and coeliac disease]. It's increasingly common that people with endo have other medical conditions, and some of them can be tied to food.

Then Eliza was diagnosed with PCOS, which causes a hormone imbalance that affects about one in ten women+. This condition is associated with increased levels of two hormones in the body: insulin and androgens, male-type hormones.

> *You can also commonly have metabolic issues as well—acne and excessive hair—those sorts of symptoms can be telltale signs. And, yeah, having that diagnosis has definitely triggered the fertility kind of thinking and conversations, because that, combined with everything else, can have an impact on your ability to get pregnant because I'm not ovulating on a necessarily regular basis. So that's something that weighs on my mind when I have previously thought about fertility as well.*

Finding a name for her pain was 'emotional, scary, but ultimately validating', but she also struggled with the reality of it all.

> *It's been something I really struggled with, this feeling that your body is self-sabotaging and the frustration that you feel like you can't control it. It's been one thing after another after another. I'm supposed to be a young person living my life unhindered by anything physical just yet. So it was really hard dealing with that. I honestly hated my body. I struggled with that for a very long time.*

Despite the challenges, as the years passed, she found these additional diagnoses a source of motivation: 'I was able to utilise my education to gain a further sense of empowerment; doing the research really helped, too.'

> *I think just with maturation, my disposition's changed a lot, too. I'm able to find gratitude and appreciate the small moments.*
>
> *I'm far more positive. I mean, it helps that I'm not as unwell as I was … However, when I am challenged by flare-ups or periods of being unwell, I kind of have the resilience—I hate that word—to get through the harder times and then really enjoy the good times in between and really make the most of them.*

Eliza advocates guided dietary change.

I have annual blood tests with my GP to ensure that everything is okay. I've been plant-based for five years now. I'm lucky not to be anaemic. I think it also correlates with you eating a lot more of a whole-foods diet. That's really, really helped as well.

She is a strong believer in the benefits of pelvic physiotherapy.

It's been a journey putting together the kind of regime that works for me and ensures I can exercise without aggravating things. That was a big challenge at first because, obviously, a lot of exercise involves activating your abs and pelvic area. With pelvic physio, I learnt how to deactivate those muscles and sense when they needed to be turned down.

After surgery, she eased back into things very gently.

I used to do lots of gentle yoga and walking and things like that, building up over time. I used to play team sports, lots of basketball. And now I have a mix of yoga, Pilates, high-intensity training and cardio, which I've found is really important. It's something that kind of jumpstarts my system as long as I don't do it too much."

Eliza is such an 'Energiser bunny', it's challenging for her to find balance. She finds that 'having a mix and not focusing too much on one muscle group or one style of exercise all the time has been key for me, then I don't aggravate things.'

She finds a correlation between food, exercise and mental health, acknowledging balance leads her to have a 'happier disposition. It also seems to reduce my flare-ups. Something about keeping things moving and not getting too stagnant helps me.'

And remember, always take the opportunity to speak to others at conferences, and anywhere, really. Look out for the most interesting people at the 'irritables' table.

Heal. Nourish. Support. Balance.

Food is fuel and promotes health and wellbeing. You can eat well to stay well, but sometimes your body needs more than you can gain from food alone.

Boost with supplements

Sometimes your body may need a boost in certain areas (vitamins and minerals) if it's not getting what it needs purely from diet. If you've ever wandered the vitamin aisle at your local supermarket, the sheer volume of available supplements can be overwhelming. Here's a list of a few to investigate.

- Zinc: This essential mineral plays a vital role in immune cell function. Zinc deficiency is associated with the development of ovarian endometrial cysts.
- Resveratrol: Found in grapes, berries and peanuts, it has exhibited anti-inflammatory, antioxidant and anti-lesion effects in endometriosis studies.
- Vitamin D: Essential for immune function, vitamin D helps modulate the immune response and promotes calcium absorption in the gut, which is essential for bone health.
- Vitamin C: Known for its antioxidant properties, vitamin C is crucial for the growth and function of immune cells. It can enhance the immune response and has been found to reduce pain symptoms in endometriosis.
- Vitamin E: This vitamin acts as an antioxidant and supports various immune functions, neutralises oxidisation and reduces pelvic pain.
- Selenium: This mineral is important for the production of antioxidant enzymes and supports the immune system, potentially reducing inflammation.
- Melatonin: This can assist as an antioxidant and anti-inflammatory, and can help manage pain, as well as insomnia. It is available over the counter for women+ aged 55 plus.

Magnesium

One supplement that deserves special attention is magnesium. Magnesium improves premenstrual tension and has been found to

Diet and nutrition **169**

reduce contractions and spasms in the fallopian tubes of women+ with endometriosis. Magnesium is also a muscle relaxant and, as a result, may affect retrograde menstruation, which we also talked about on page 13 as a cause of endometriosis. It also helps with migraines.

Essential for regulating certain hormones, it can help calm the brain and promote relaxation. This includes gamma-aminobutyric acid (GABA), an inhibitory neurotransmitter (chemical messenger) that helps to reduce anxiety.

It supports nerve signalling, which impacts pain. Magnesium also assists with protein metabolism, healthy cell division, protecting against DNA damage, the regulation of blood pressure and blood sugar, and bone development. It is so important for women+, especially those taking hormone suppression medications, like the pill.

Known to have laxative properties, it helps you poo; it softens stools and helps bowel movements to pass more easily. In addition, magnesium relaxes the intestinal muscles, which assists in establishing a smoother rhythm for passing stools and it eases constipation.

A recent study also found magnesium supports folate levels, a vitamin B that helps support healthy baby development in pregnancy. It also suggested that taking vitamin B12 and magnesium is important for healthy ageing and avoiding neurodegenerative diseases such as Parkinson's and Alzheimer's disease. It really is an essential mineral.

There are multiple ways you can increase your magnesium intake:
- Eat it: You can find it in green leafy vegetables such as spinach, legumes, nuts, seeds and whole grains.
- Drink it in mineral water, but look at the milligram-to-litre ratio, around 50 mg is best.
- Mix it as a supplement powder.
- Take it as a vitamin tablet.
- Soak in it: cheap Epsom salts are great in the bath.
- Rub it in: Magnesium oil is a combination of chloride flakes and water; it has an oily feel, but it isn't technically an oil.

Be aware

Food is medicine, and nourishing your body and brain is fundamental to wellbeing and mood. It can help avoid the *hangry* and the *paingry* negative emotions. You may not be able to stop endometriosis, but you can take positive steps to reduce painful symptoms, pelvic pain and gut-wrenching toileting challenges as well as improve your energy levels.

So take positive steps to change what you can in your endo life, and we hope it makes a positive difference. Visit Nutritionfacts.org (nutritionfacts.org/topics/) to learn more about the impacts of foods on your body.

Be prepared

Any dramatic change in your diet will have a big impact on your appetite, stomach, bowel, wind and toileting. Please speak to your GP and get a referral to a dietitian. Don't follow fad diets—all they do is eliminate the nutrients.

The information provided in this chapter and the book has been researched, but we are not dietitians, nutritionists, doctors or experts in any way. We are on our own health journeys and have shared some of what we have learnt.

Diet and nutrition **171**

CHAPTER 13
Exercise for endo

For individuals with endometriosis, engaging in certain types of exercise can help manage symptoms and improve overall wellbeing. It's important to choose exercises that do not exacerbate pain or discomfort. Here are some of the best exercises recommended for endometriosis.

- Walking is a gentle, low-impact exercise that can help reduce stress and improve cardiovascular health without putting too much strain on the pelvic area.
- Swimming offers a full-body workout that minimises impact on the joints and pelvic area, making it an excellent choice for those with endometriosis. You can dog paddle like Ellie Angel-Mobbs (see page 187) or race like Emily Seebohm.
- Yoga is beneficial in alleviating pelvic pain. It helps manage endometriosis by improving breathing patterns and posture, and decreasing pain from everyday activities. Child's pose, supine spinal twist and happy baby pose are among the recommended poses that can help ease endo pain by gently stretching and relaxing the pelvic muscles (see page 176 for some stretches that can help).
- Pilates focuses on strengthening the core and pelvic floor muscles, but it is not helpful to those with pelvic floor tension who need to relax, not tighten. It emphasises controlled movements and breathing, which can help in managing pain and improving muscle function. Just try before you commit.

- Exercises that focus on posture correcting, diaphragmatic breathing, lunges, squats, relaxation, muscle awareness and stretches for back and pelvic floor muscles can be helpful. Aimed at building strength, especially in the lower back and core, they can improve posture and support the pelvic area. Exercises like glute bridges, bird dogs and squats with chair assistance are beneficial.

Rolling with life's curveballs: Lisa's story

We met Lisa earlier in the osteopathy section. I have been seeing Dr Lisa Gadd for about ten years after recovering from a virus that left me with foreign pain and fatigue. She has even helped my 'Gracie' shoulder, injured while feeding my granddaughter with a bottle — she loved flinging herself backwards (her other Nana has the same injury). I find her treatment both relieving and strengthening. She always has something in her toolbox to help with pain from fibromyalgia and arthritis.

At around the same time I met her, Lisa was recovering from a major stroke caused by a brain bleed, and doctors believe it was caused by the medication she was taking to manage her endometriosis: the common contraceptive pill. The extremely fit and active 24-year-old spent three months in and out of the hospital and needed to re-learn how to walk and talk properly. She couldn't drive and left her job to recover.

As an endo warrior, she was already resilient and, post-stroke, she has learnt how to rebuild the mind, body and spirit after trauma. This made her even more committed to supporting others, and she started Living Health Group, offering osteopathy and remedial massage services.

From her early teenage years, Lisa suffered from heavy, painful periods, and her GP prescribed the pill when Lisa was 20 years of age. As a result of the stroke four years later, she has been advised not to resume synthetic hormone treatment, including the pill.

Lisa feels incredibly frustrated to be unable to have hormonal treatments and is also limited with medications she can have because of her risk of stroke. 'As an endo warrior, I still have daily challenges, living in daily pain and constant fatigue.'

As a health practitioner, Lisa follows her own advice:

> *I aim to keep myself fit and healthy — I exercise daily, supplement daily and aim for nine hours of sleep a day. I try to manage my stress as best I can, which can be difficult when you run your own business and have staff to look after and manage.*
>
> *I've had allergy testing done to know what foods to avoid my gut from flaring up. I do daily breathing exercises and journalling to help manage stress.*

Lisa shares that she has 'an incredibly supportive partner, family and friends around me that help'. She notes: 'Financially, endo is a burden: constant GP or specialist visits, scans or hospital bills, days off work — and when you work for yourself, there is no such thing as sick leave.'

The week of our interview, Lisa had spent time in the hospital with pneumonia after soldiering on with no voice to keep her patient appointments. Some days she experiences such excruciating pain that she is in greater need than the person she's treating. 'I have been to the hospital three times with lower right quadrant abdominal pain, which the doctors dismiss as having anything to do with my endo', and this makes her feel 'invalidated'.

Lisa finds pain medication 'has side effects on my gut, so I opt for a heat pack or TENS machine where possible'. Lisa wants to raise awareness that 'periods are not meant to be painful. Find a practitioner who listens — it's okay to change practitioners, be they GPs, specialists, or allied health.'

She feels she is 'even more empathetic with my patients, understanding the implications of what it is to lose bodily function, to deal with the emotional loss of poor health' as a result of the stroke and living with endometriosis.

Lisa harnessed courage and a firm commitment to reframe her belief systems to ensure she came back stronger than ever. In doing so, she developed a new level of understanding for the clients she was working with as a health practitioner and coach.

> *During my five-year osteopathic degree, I also worked as a personal training and group fitness instructor, working with many runners and triathletes.*

Exercise for endo **175**

I've since managed to complete a few sprint and Olympic distance triathlons. In March 2024, I wanted to really challenge myself and strive for a 70.3 (half ironman)—this involved a 1.9-kilometre ocean swim, a 90-kilometre ride, followed by a 21-kilometre run... Training for a 70.3 with endo isn't easy, but it teaches me a valuable lesson to listen to my body.

On days I physically can't train either at all or at the level I hope to, that's ok. I have to keep reminding myself of progress over progression.

Sometimes, not everything goes to plan; recently, I was building for my second 70.3 half ironman on the Sunshine Coast. My progress was going well, and I was fairly consistent with training. I had been experiencing some terrible endo flare-ups. However, three weeks out from the race, I ended up with pneumonia, stopping any training for two weeks. Things don't always go to plan, but I readjust, refocus and go again. Now, to look forward to what is next.

Dr Lisa Gadd's endometriosis stretches to attain 'living health'

Exercise and stretching can be very beneficial for managing the symptoms of endometriosis, particularly by helping to reduce pain, improve flexibility and alleviate muscle tension. Here are ten specific exercises and stretches that may help.

Child's pose (Balasana)

Benefits: Stretches the lower back, hips and thighs, promoting relaxation and easing pelvic pain.

How to do it: Kneel on the floor, sit back on your heels, and reach your arms forward as you lower your torso towards the floor. Rest your forehead on the mat and hold the position for one to two minutes, breathing deeply.

Cat-cow stretch

Benefits: Mobilises the spine, stretches the back and abdomen, and helps relieve pelvic tension.

How to do it: Start on your hands and knees in a tabletop position. Inhale as you arch your back (cow pose), lifting your head and tailbone. Exhale as you round your spine (cat pose), tucking your chin and tailbone. Repeat for one to two minutes, moving with your breath.

Pelvic tilts

Benefits: Strengthens the pelvic floor muscles and lower back, improving core stability and reducing pelvic pain.

How to do it: Lie on your back with your knees bent and feet flat on the floor. Gently tilt your pelvis upward, flattening your lower back against the floor. Hold for a few seconds, then release. Repeat 10 to 15 times.

Knee-to-chest stretch

Benefits: Stretches the lower back and hips, relieving tension in the pelvic region.

How to do it: Lie on your back with your knees bent. Draw one knee towards your chest, holding it with both hands. Keep the opposite foot on the floor or extend the leg straight for a deeper stretch. Hold for 20 to 30 seconds, then switch legs.

Reclined bound angle pose (Supta Baddha Konasana)

Benefits: Opens the hips and pelvis, reduces groin and lower abdomen tension, and promotes relaxation.

How to do it: Lie on your back and bring the soles of your feet together, allowing your knees to fall open to the sides. Place your arms at your sides or on your belly. Hold for one to two minutes, focusing on deep, relaxed breathing.

Seated forward bend (Paschimottanasana)

Benefits: Stretches the lower back, hamstrings and pelvic region, helping to relieve tension and pain.

How to do it: Sit with your legs extended straight in front of you. Inhale and lengthen your spine, then exhale as you reach forward, hinging at the hips. Hold your feet or shins, and stay in the stretch for 30 to 60 seconds.

Hip flexor stretch

Benefits: Stretches the hip flexors, which can become tight and contribute to pelvic pain.

How to do it: Start in a lunge position with one foot forward and the other knee on the ground behind you. Gently push your hips forward, feeling a stretch in the front of your hip. Hold for 20 to 30 seconds, then switch sides.

Pigeon pose (Eka Pada Rajakapotasana)

Benefits: Deeply stretches the hips and glutes, which can relieve tension in the pelvic region.

How to do it: Start in a tabletop position, then bring one knee towards your wrist. Extend the opposite leg straight back. Lower your hips towards the floor, keeping them square. Hold for one to two minutes, then switch sides.

Bridge pose (Setu Bandhasana)

Benefits: Strengthens the core, glutes and pelvic floor while stretching the chest and spine.

How to do it: Lie on your back with your knees bent and feet hip-width apart. Press into your feet and lift your hips towards the ceiling, squeezing your glutes. Hold for 20 to 30 seconds, then slowly lower down. Repeat five to ten times.

Butterfly stretch

Benefits: Stretches the inner thighs and hips, relieving tension in the pelvic area.

How to do it: Sit with your feet together and knees bent out to the sides. Hold your feet with your hands, and gently press your knees towards the floor with your elbows. Hold the stretch for 30 to 60 seconds.

Lisa says:

These exercises and stretches can be incorporated into a daily routine to help manage the symptoms of endometriosis. Remember to listen to your body and adjust or skip any movements that cause discomfort. Working with a physical therapist or yoga instructor with experience managing pelvic pain may also be helpful.

Protecting with abdominal exercises

It's advisable to avoid high-impact exercises and intense abdominal workouts, such as running, burpees, box jumps or crunches, as they can stress the lower back and abdominal wall, potentially worsening endometriosis symptoms.

It's important to listen to your body and modify exercises as needed. If an exercise causes pain or discomfort, avoiding it and trying a different activity is best. Many exercises have modifications that may be more comfortable.

Be aware

Engaging in regular physical activity, even if it's just a little movement each day, can contribute to effective management of your endometriosis symptoms. It also helps your mental health, empowering you to take charge of your body.

Be prepared

Before starting any new exercise regimen, it's recommended to consult with a healthcare provider, especially if you have severe symptoms. A physical therapist, especially one specialising in women+'s health or pelvic floor rehabilitation, can provide personalised advice and guidance.

Raising period and endo awareness: Kayla's story

Kayla Itsines, co-founder of Sweat, exudes an energy that is electrifying and inspiring. Her fitness empire started with her running training sessions in her parent's backyard (her dad even built a roof for her boot camp clients). The Sweat app, which she co-founded in 2015, has had more than 30 million downloads, while her personal Instagram following (at the time of writing) is approaching 16 million—four million more than the entire number of Aussies on the social media platform.

Yet behind the bubbly, motivated persona exists a young woman who's experienced debilitating pain and all of the typical endometriosis symptoms since she first started menstruating at the age of 12. She recalls many times when she was sent home from school and couldn't take part in her beloved sport, and a horrifying fall downstairs at school when pain suddenly made her 'double over', which was embarrassing for a girl who prides herself on being 'a really coordinated person'.

Kayla is now 'at pains' to raise awareness.

I grappled with debilitating cramps, nausea and heavy bleeding every month. It felt like my periods were getting progressively more painful. What used to be several excruciating but bearable days each month turned into cancelling plans with friends and family and missing work. When my period arrived, all I could do was lie in bed and wait for it to be over.

I think one of the biggest things that people do not understand is that period pains and being in debilitating pain is just not normal. I was walking around with a heat pack every single day during school; students and teachers would know me for having a heat pack down my jumper.

I used to be in awe of my friends who were able to play netball on their period—to me, that was unimaginable. I would never be able to play sports and have my period at the same time. Not only was I getting pain during my period, but I was getting pain during my ovulation. But I didn't have a period tracking app back in the day. I didn't know when I was ovulating. I didn't know why I was suddenly in pain when I was nowhere near my period.

Kayla recalls trying to explain her pain to teachers:

> *I had male physical education teachers, and I was saying, 'I don't want to do this. I love sport. I'm just in so much pain.' They're like, 'you can play'.*
>
> *One of my most traumatic moments was during a swimming carnival. I honestly feel sick telling this story. I had my period, and one of the male teachers called out on a microphone, 'Kayla, you're up next.' Despite being very confident as a kid, I said, 'I can't; I have my period'. And he yelled through a microphone, 'Kayla, shove a tampon up there and get in the water'. Everyone laughed, and it was so embarrassing.*

Kayla is deeply grateful that her mum, who is also a teacher, understood her pain and 100 per cent supported her.

> *I'm lucky my mum was so understanding. Every single female above my age (33) in my family has had a hysterectomy. Now, whether they knew they had endometriosis or not, we don't know ... but I'm fearful I am next for a hysterectomy, and I hate that, I really hate that worry.*

When Kayla was recommended for laparoscopic surgery, she felt validated to have a 'name for her pain' but being told by the surgeon 'that I might not be able to have kids was scary and upsetting for a long time, until I had children'. She says the hardest thing about endo is 'knowing that no matter what you do, it won't ever go away'.

> *I also hate that endo doesn't discriminate. It doesn't say, 'Look, you don't drink alcohol. You don't take drugs. You don't smoke.' I am this perfectly healthy human who is the epitome of health and fitness, yet I have endo. In a way, though, I see it as a blessing as well because my voice has given a voice to so many other women. The fact that I have it, that I have been able to show I manage it, also that I was able to have kids as well has given so many women the confidence to come forward and speak up about their endo symptoms—not only come forward but go get checked, go to the doctor, go get the surgery even.*

I have been really honest about that surgery. It is hard recovering from any surgery, but for endo I need six weeks off. I always say I'd rather have a caesarean than have that surgery. However, just like having a baby, it's better at the other end. So, it's hard, but it's, honestly, helped so much.

In the lead-up to her second surgery, knowing what was coming, Kayla felt better prepared, but still quite fearful and anxious. Her daily life, even just the snippets shared on socials, is running around with the two kids, balancing the children, family life, work and travel, and she is often forced to accept that her body needs that time to rest and recover. She lives with the knowledge that, despite her schedule, when the pain from endometriosis symptoms strike, she is 'stuck in bed', which is the opposite to how the world sees the unbelievably physically active Kayla in exercise videos.

That is why sharing her story and that endo doesn't discriminate has been such an important message for younger women+ particularly, not just her followers and subscribers, but for the whole community. Kayla's honesty about vulnerability has inspired so many.

One of my biggest regrets was not coming forward and telling people about my endometriosis earlier. The reason I didn't do that is because I was told by a male doctor to get ready and be prepared to not be able to have kids. So, when I was told that, I hid my endometriosis diagnosis for so long.

In 2018, Kayla was 'over the moon' to learn she was pregnant: 'I remember feeling the most enormous sense of gratitude to my body for supporting me despite my endometriosis struggles.'

Kayla was devastated when her endo symptoms returned with a vengeance after her daughter was born, experiencing 'low blood pressure, blood clots, pain in my legs and my lower back, and I was unable to leave bed for the first two days of my period'.

For the first time, she experienced painful cysts and collapsed while filming a workout. In the hospital emergency department, she underwent tests and ultrasounds and found multiple cysts on her ovaries. One had ruptured, which means fluid and blood from the cyst go into the abdomen.

Kayla was advised to avoid any high-intensity exercise, which deflated her and made her concerned about managing her professional commitments. She says she felt an 'overwhelming sense of guilt' and felt defeated by her own body. She struggled to do basic workouts and grappled with the lack of control she had over her own body, feeling her sense of self and her body weren't coordinated.

In the six months following the debilitating flare-up, Kayla suffered another four burst cysts, which were not only excruciatingly painful but life-threatening, necessitating a second endo-laparoscopic surgery.

Kalya told the surgeon she wanted 'fewer scars' because she was concerned for her reputation as the 'Queen of Abs'.

I said to the doctor, 'I don't want you to put cuts all over me. I don't want to be covered in scars because I'm showing my stomach all the time.' This is me being really vain. So, they said, 'No worries. We'll put all the tools into your belly button. We do one incision.' So, they put nine tools or whatever it is through my belly button.

Unfortunately, an infection resulted in her needing further surgery, leaving her with 'a scar for a belly button'.

After her first surgery, she knew she needed the full six weeks to heal, but this time, she also had a toddler. She is grateful to her close family, who helped her recover physically and maintain a positive outlook. 'I love to work out, and training people is my job, but I just need to accept stepping back is crucial for my body to heal.' While studies show gentle exercise can help manage endometriosis symptoms, recovering from surgery requires time and patience.

She chose to share her experience with surgery and recovery to inform and empower others and help to remove the stigma.

I remember, before my first surgery, I searched the internet to learn more. There was so little information and even fewer personal stories shared. It just made me feel even more alone and overwhelmed.

There is still such stigma around symptoms; it is taboo. I thought: 'What I am living with is not rare—so why aren't people talking about it?' Girls and women need to know about endometriosis, where to get help and how to live with it. Being told there is no cure is so distressing. By speaking out, I hope to help others so they can learn endo is not the end of the world. There are ways to manage symptoms, and they can achieve their best healthy selves.

Like all endo warriors, she has experienced feelings of guilt, anger at helplessness, fear of missing out and regret for letting people down. For Kayla, these stressors are amplified. She has employees, deadlines for content, children to care for and a self-imposed high bar to achieve. By acknowledging the hard conversations and doubts internally and dealing with them in a positive way, she strives to manage her expectations of herself.

Kayla was thrilled to learn she was pregnant again, and Jax was born in January 2023. Kayla needed a caesarean section, as she had with Arna. With two endometriosis surgeries under her belt, she waited six weeks for the all clear from her doctor before she would 'even think about training again'.

During her recovery period, she shared uplifting posts on social media, letting followers know it is important to share personal feelings of uncertainty, insecurity and fear. She expressed her concerns about the impact of pregnancy, nurturing leave and 'time out' for endometriosis on both her body and her business.

Kayla is already making sure her daughter Arna is aware of the symptoms she sees her mum experience. She is hopeful science finds any hereditary link before Arna starts menstruating, and a cure will be discovered and available soon.

> *I'm so, so concerned for my daughter, obviously knowing there is a genetic link, knowing that my grandma, my mum, me, my cousins, a lot of us have it, makes me very concerned about being educated and understanding the symptoms.*
>
> *In my experience, burning the endo, cutting the endo, whatever they do to get that out is not minimally invasive. I get burned, I get cut, I get everything. And then I wake up and I'm in pain because I've had a huge surgery that requires six weeks off, not one week. And then I have people who have come to me say, 'Kayla, I'm so scared, I've got endo, I've got to have surgery. I don't want six weeks off.' My advice is that the six weeks off will help you have no weeks off in the future rather than constantly being in pain month after month during your ovulation and during a period ... it is so worth it. Take the six weeks off. If you calculate the amount of time that we have off with endo, it's way more than six weeks, way more.*

She relates how financially and physically hard it is for most women+ to take time off from work and get help if they have children. 'I understand that is extremely difficult. The thing that I will say is I will never lie about how much help I have.'

Kayla, unsurprisingly, doesn't 'do' rest very well.

> *The six weeks is active recovery for me. It's not sitting down on a couch doing absolutely nothing. When I wake from the surgery, I try to move my arms a little bit to try to get rid of that gas pain. I don't do anything with my core. I'm just sitting down, trying to move my arms around when I can. I get on a treadmill, but I'm walking at 3 kilometres an hour, like one foot after the other, just trying to remove the gas in my body.*
>
> *And then all I will do for six weeks is walk. And then once I get clearance from my doctor, which is probably around*

four and a half weeks in, they'll clear me for some upper body training. I get guided help with this, with a physiotherapist, but my core feels completely mashed up and wrecked.

Even once cleared to train ... you don't feel normal, even at the six-week mark. Like you're cleared to train, but you still feel like 'what just happened to my insides?' So, I don't know if it takes a good three months to get back into training, but once you're back into training, you feel wonderful.

Kayla shares her 'endo exercise' regime: 'I now have the program in the app, and you can use it post-op, when you're pregnant, after birth, recovering from a caesarean.' There's also a low-impact option: 'When you have endo, and you're having a flare-up, the last thing you want to do is start jumping around because you get so lightheaded and you're in so much pain.'

Kayla shares that she 'honestly hates endo. I hate it for so many reasons. I hate it because you do nothing wrong. My health is my life's mission, no drinking, I've never done a drug, never smoked in my life.'

Sometimes, when you're in pain, not sleeping well, and feeling in low energy, it can impact your self-esteem to see high-profile, active, and busy endo warriors like Kayla. Everyone is different, and as she explains, you don't see her downtime. You can start building your own fitness, and follow the link to endo exercises in the references and through the Sweat app.

CHAPTER 14

Rest and recuperation

'R&R' is a common term. It can mean 'rest and recuperation, 'rest and relaxation' or 'rest and recreation'. The primary word is *rest*, which according to the Australian Oxford Dictionary means to 'cease work or movement in order to relax, sleep, or recover strength'.

The best kinds of medicine are free, and the seven doctors of nature are exercise, water, sun, fresh air, healthy food, laughter and sleep.

Listening to what your body needs: Ellie's story

Award-winning radio announcer and endo warrior Ellie Angel-Mobbs struggled for 12 years without a diagnosis for her endo. She has been using her voice and empowering others about the disease since 2016, sharing her battles with the physical, fertility and mental challenges.

> *There are days when I do come to work and I am on the studio floor, just lying down with my hot water bottle, trying to get through that pain. It is what it is, and I'm very blessed to do what I do every single day. It's about putting one foot in front of the other. It can be the simplest of goals, like making yourself a cup of tea or making the bed on those bad days, and not beating yourself up as well when you're unable to achieve those things.*
>
> *I love bushwalking. I love going out, and when the sun's out, I'm out. I love my vitamin D. I've got a Fitbit. I do my 10000 steps every single day. If I'm having one of those days where I can feel the*

pain getting worse and worse and worse, I'll just have a little walk around the block ... The walking does help, especially because I get nerve pain down my legs from the adhesions. I love swimming, too. In summer, I go to the local council swimming pool, and I do dog paddle. There's nothing graceful about it, but I find it therapeutic as well because of its low impact on the body.

If my body is not up to it, I've learned that when it says no, it means no. I need to rest. I have anaemia with low iron as well. I take iron supplements and I get regular iron infusions as well. Probably every second night, I'll have a broken sleep where I will wake up in that physical pain to the point where sometimes I sleep with a bucket next to me because the pain will be so horrific that I will start vomiting. My poor husband will be next to me, and he knows the drill — 'There's nothing I can do. I'll hold Ellie's hair back'.

That's a big relationship test, but sleep is also very important. Everything will be thrown out if you don't get a good night's sleep. I started seeing a pain specialist, and her number one thing was, 'We're going to get on top of this pain at night, and we're going to get your sleep to be magnificent.'

Fatigue and Spoon Theory

We know that fatigue and managing pain make you feel like you're meandering aimlessly through life, dictated by the flares inflicted by endometriosis and other conditions. Chronic conditions are challenging, and while I don't personally share your journey with endo, I have other lived experiences with other invisible conditions.

I recall going to an exercise physiologist after a nasty virus in 2014 left me exhausted and in pain. My expectation was that the therapist would 'fix' me and restore my previous fitness levels.

I was told to consider what I thought of as mundane, routine, normal 'stuff' around the house as reasonable and achievable goals — things like unloading the dishwasher, going to the mailbox, cooking a meal and even showering. I left in tears and called my husband from the car, complaining about what a waste of money it was.

I remember him gently reminding me that those simple tasks I mentioned were often beyond my capacity. I needed help from my mum to manage the boring stuff that, in the past, wasn't even on my radar; I simply did what needed to be done, pottering and multitasking without thought…until I couldn't even gather the energy to get myself lunch, let alone shop and cook for my family.

I was told I had chronic fatigue (ME/CFS), which I am embarrassed to say I hadn't considered a real illness. I can attest it is disabling and profound. We are now seeing many people post-COVID-19 suffering from the same symptoms I had. In fact, according to Yale University, about half of those diagnosed with long COVID meet the diagnostic criteria for ME/CFS.

I was introduced to Spoon Theory, developed by Christine Miserandino in 2013, to pace my energy levels, and it really allowed me to forgive myself for my lagging energy. It starts with the premise that you have 12 spoons of energy per day. You take one spoon away if you didn't sleep well the night before, if you didn't eat properly or skipped your medicine or vitamins. If you were sick with a cold, that would deplete your energy to the equivalent of four spoons.

As a guide, one spoon is the energy you would use to get out of bed, get dressed or watch TV. Two spoons are the energy to bathe, style your hair, get on the computer, read or study. Three spoons are the effort it takes to make a meal, make plans and socialise with your friends, do some light housework or drive somewhere, say, to get the kids from school. Four spoons is what it takes to go to school or work, do the shopping and exercise.

Having a finite number of spoons makes you prioritise your tasks for the day. With only 12 spoons, you really start to think about what you use them for. It can also be a signal that you are doing too much if you find yourself with only a few spoons at any point in your day.

It is so heavy carrying a chronic illness, particularly pain. What I've learned is to allow myself the time I need to manage my health and to try not to be angry, negative, frustrated or sad about the limitations of my body because that is a waste of the precious energy I have. Don't compare yourself to anyone else. Be alert to signs you need to wash your spoons and rest or chances are, you'll crash.

Finding a creative outlet: Jess's story

Jess Coldrey has channelled her lived experience with endometriosis into various art forms. She went to school with my daughter Brianna, who recalls they were often in the toilets at the same time but weren't aware they were each struggling with similar symptoms of pain and heavy menstrual bleeding. They also did both visual arts and communication and they would display their works together.

Jess is the global partner engagement lead for the World Green Building Council and has earned a Bachelor of Arts in Human Geography and a Bachelor of Fine Arts, and is currently studying for a Master of Science in Humanitarian Engineering with Management at the University of Warwick, England.

I saw Jess's art displayed at a Hudson Institute of Medical Research event, and I was blown away by the most vibrant, beautiful expression of feeling I've ever seen. She experienced endo symptoms from her early teens and had her first laparoscopic surgery in 2021. She decided to channel her physical experiences into her artistic expression of the pain, the surreal twilight of coming out of an anaesthetic, and visualisation of invasive endometriosis lesions growing unabated.

Thinking about making some art series about my experience brought me meaning and purpose around what I'd been through.

Initially, my inspiration was in thinking about the diagnosis process. I was interested in how I'd previously tried to talk to GPs, what kind of words I would use to describe my pain, and perhaps how words hadn't been enough. Then, I started exploring photography, robotics and fashion as ways to express different symptoms and a personal experience of trying to communicate pain and the sort of performative elements I saw. Inspired, I worked on a series of hospital gowns while I was living in France.

I was really inspired by working in France and how Endo France approaches their advocacy, which is trying to create a sense of curiosity, dignity and beauty, which I think is a lot different to other approaches in endo advocacy, which is more focused on pain, all confronting and scary elements.

I wanted to play more with that vibrant, colourful language, to try and inspire people who would otherwise look away to look a bit deeper and to ask a few more questions. From there, I started to create some textile work. I thought using pillows, cushions, quilts and pyjamas I'd worn in hospital would channel this. I used an AI [artificial intelligence] surreal landscape that represented my experience of navigating endo.

Part of the journey with endo involves trying a lot of different medications, and they can have different effects on how we feel and how we sense our surroundings. I try to use other ways to deal with the pain in a way that's more manageable day to day.

I think that impacted my explorations, that disassociating, the feeling that I'm disconnecting from my body when I'm in pain. It's the way the brain can sometimes cope with extreme circumstances. So, inspired by my laparoscopic surgery, I created a dream-like aesthetic using my quilts.

My mum had bought me these pyjamas for surgery. They were unbuttoned so I wouldn't have to put anything over my head, and they had little rabbits and woodland creatures on them. They were so cute, and they wove into this dream I was having while I was in surgery. The rabbits were jumping around in my mind. I guess that symbolised fertility; they were multiplying and turning into these dandelions floating around the world, and soon enough, the whole world was full of them ... I wanted to play with that sensitisation and re-navigate a familiar landscape that felt alien and unfamiliar, like my sense of self, with these new bodily feelings after surgery.

I still struggle with endo pain every day. I'm a private person, so I express myself through my art. I am getting better at communicating. I do retreat into myself sometimes, but I can communicate more with what I'm feeling and say to colleagues at work, 'I'm having a bit of a flare-up now; if I look out of it or I give you a strange look, don't take it personally'.

I might say that I'm just going to sit here and try and listen into the meeting, and maybe, maybe, I'll send some thoughts afterwards, and we'll catch up about it later. I have learnt that awareness of what's going on and having boundaries gives you a safe space to speak up and share your symptoms.

Cold therapy

People in cold climates like Scandinavia, Japan, Russia and Canada have been practising cold water therapy for centuries. The temperature range for cold therapy is between 10 and 15 degrees Celsius.

For years, I have been finishing my showers with cold water, and I breathe into it to minimise the big gulp of air my sympathetic nervous system automatically takes from the shock. Sometimes, it seems as if a couple of minutes is an hour, but other times, it is so refreshing that I linger longer.

I find this really helps with pain and inflammation and clears my mind.

Benefits of cold water therapy

Cold water therapy has a range of benefits that can also be used to help manage endometriosis symptoms.

- Reduced inflammation and muscle soreness: Cold water immersion effectively minimises inflammation and muscle soreness. Exposure to cold causes vasoconstriction, which reduces blood flow to muscles and helps decrease swelling and lactic acid accumulation. This is particularly beneficial for athletes recovering from intense workouts.
- Enhanced muscle recovery: Cold water therapy can accelerate recovery by promoting muscle repair and reducing tissue damage. The cold temperature helps to alleviate oxidative stress and swelling, allowing individuals to bounce back more quickly after physical exertion.
- Pain relief: Cold exposure has been linked to the release of endorphins, the body's natural pain-relieving chemicals. Endorphins can help block pain signals and promote a sense of

wellbeing, which may be beneficial for managing endometriosis pain. Some research suggests that cold exposure may modulate brain and spinal cord pain pathways. By altering the way the body perceives and processes pain, cold immersion may help reduce the intensity of endometriosis-related pain.

- Psychological benefits: Cold exposure has been shown to reduce stress and anxiety. Endometriosis can be a significant source of stress and anxiety for those who suffer from it. Cold immersion may indirectly relieve pain by promoting relaxation and reducing stress levels. While more research is needed to fully understand the mechanisms by which cold immersion can help with endometriosis pain, these potential benefits suggest that it may be a valuable complementary therapy for those seeking relief from this condition.
- Boosted immune function: Some studies suggest that cold water exposure can enhance immune response by increasing the production of white blood cells, which are crucial for fighting infections. This may help individuals become more resilient against common illnesses.
- Increased circulation: Cold exposure followed by rewarming can enhance circulation. When you exit cold water, blood vessels dilate, improving blood flow and cardiovascular health.
- Metabolic benefits: Cold water immersion may temporarily increase metabolic rate, potentially aiding in weight management and fat loss. This is because the body needs more energy to maintain its core temperature after exposure to cold.
- Stress reduction and improved sleep: Cold water therapy can induce a relaxation response, lowering heart rate and blood pressure, which can help reduce stress and promote better sleep quality.

Cold therapy practice

Cold therapy is a practice that involves using cold, hard nature to help gain control over physiological functions such as breathing, heart rate, and blood circulation. The Wim Hof technique is built upon three fundamental components: breathing exercises, cold exposure and mental commitment. When combined, these elements are believed to reduce stress, support a stronger immune system, increase energy, improve sleep and enhance physical performance.

Cold shower at home

You can try cold water therapy at home, and here are some practical tips to get started:

Note that the first 15 or so seconds are always the hardest. Your skin will react to the sudden drop in temperature, and you may feel an intense urge to return to warmth. During this time, your breathing may quicken instinctively, contributing to distress. Focus on controlling your breath to stay calm.

The optimal amount of cold exposure is about ten minutes per week. You can break this into daily sessions of one to two minutes per day to get the optimal benefits.

Cold therapy for endometriosis research at The University of Adelaide

Cold therapy is currently being investigated for its potential benefits in alleviating symptoms of endometriosis. A pilot study at The University of Adelaide, supported by a philanthropic gift from the Wilson Foundation, is exploring cold therapy's efficacy in managing endometriosis symptoms. The research aims to gather data over a 12-month period to objectively quantify the molecular and cellular effects on various factors, including:

- pelvic pain intensity
- psychological wellbeing
- characteristics of endometriosis lesions
- responses from the autonomic nervous system and endocrine system
- innate immune responses.

The lead researcher, Professor Mark Hutchinson, noted that, if effective, cold therapy could offer a new, natural treatment option for many women+ who have not found relief through traditional methods such as medication or surgery.

Cold plunges are considered a stressor, but learning to control the body's response can bring potential health benefits through what is termed 'learned optimism'. However, sensitivity to cold water can vary significantly, and it is important to gradually increase tolerance, beginning with short immersions and progressing to longer times as your capacity develops.

While the formal research is ongoing, there is an accumulating number of reports from women+ who have found relief from endometriosis symptoms through cold therapy. Many practitioners report improvements in pain management and overall wellbeing, suggesting that combining cold exposure and controlled breathing may help modulate pain perception and enhance mood.

Safety precautions

Pregnant individuals should avoid extreme temperatures. If you have heart problems, circulatory issues, high blood pressure or autoimmune disorders, use extreme caution, and always have someone with you in case of an adverse reaction—including uncontrolled dysregulation of breathing reflexes. Call an ambulance if you experience arrhythmias or if the person you're with loses consciousness.

Be aware

In the context of cold plunge pools, keep your neck and head out of the water. You may feel numb, heavy or wobbly when exiting a cold plunge pool, so proceed cautiously and, ideally, have someone with you for support.

Be prepared

Royal Lifesaving Australia warns of cold water shock: as your heart rate rises, blood vessels in your skin rapidly begin to close, making blood flow challenging. Watch out for signs such as rapid and uncontrolled breathing patterns, hyperventilation, confusion, loss of coordination, body rigidity, or fatigue. Seek medical attention if these symptoms occur.

Heat therapy

Heat therapy, also known as thermotherapy, is commonly used by individuals with endometriosis to help alleviate pain and discomfort associated with the condition. Here's how heat therapy can be beneficial for managing endometriosis pain.

- Increased circulation: Heat therapy promotes blood flow to the affected areas, which can help deliver oxygen and nutrients necessary for healing and reduce muscle tension.
- Muscle relaxation: Applying heat can relax the muscles in the pelvic region, which may help relieve cramping and spasms associated with endometriosis.
- Pain relief: Heat can affect pain receptors in the body, potentially reducing the perception of pain. This analgesic effect can be particularly helpful during menstrual cramps or flare-ups.
- Stress reduction: The soothing effect of heat can lead to relaxation and a reduction in stress levels, which may indirectly contribute to pain relief. Stress can exacerbate pain, so managing it is crucial for those with chronic conditions like endometriosis.
  Heat therapy can be applied in various forms, including:
- moist heat: warm baths, warm wet towels or moist heating packs that you microwave; moist heat often penetrates deeper and may be more effective for some individuals
- dry heat: electric heating pads or dry heating packs; while effective, dry heat may not penetrate as deeply as moist heat.

Usage considerations

While many women+ report positive effects from heat therapy, it is not universally effective for everyone. It's important to experiment with different methods to find what works best for you.

- Duration and safety: It's essential to follow recommended guidelines for duration to avoid burns or skin irritation; for instance, direct heat applications should typically be limited to 20 minutes, while warm baths can be enjoyed for longer periods.
- Consultation with healthcare providers: Before starting heat therapy, consult with your healthcare provider to ensure it is appropriate for your specific situation and to determine the best methods.

Be aware

Heat therapy can be a valuable self-management strategy for many women+ with endometriosis, helping to alleviate pain and improve quality of life. While it may not be effective for everyone, its benefits in increasing circulation, relaxing muscles and reducing pain perception make it a commonly recommended complementary treatment option for managing endometriosis symptoms.

Be prepared

Hot water bottle injuries are a serious and common issue, often leading to burns that require extensive medical care. These injuries are frequent causes of preventable burns, with many cases necessitating hospital admission and even skin grafts due to the severity.

Common risks include the hot water splashing or overflowing as you fill the bottle, the bottle rupturing or bursting and *erythema ab igne*, burns and lesions on the skin caused by repeated exposure to low-level heat over the same location, often found on the pelvic areas of those living with endometriosis. You can limit the risks by regularly replacing the hot water bottle, not using boiling water to fill it, and avoiding overfilling or putting pressure on the bottle.

Fabric-covered wheat bags (including wrap-around Velcro types), infrared, TENS and other battery-operated heat packs are all alternatives, and should only be used as per the manufacturer's instructions.

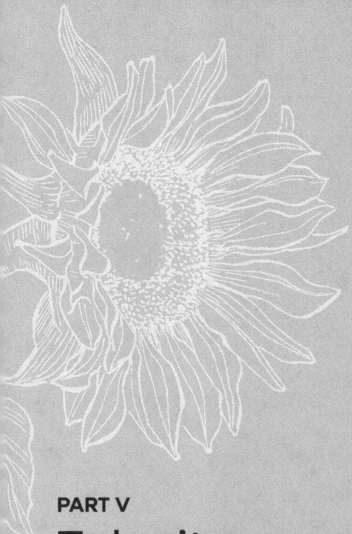

PART V
Take it on
Know your rights

CHAPTER 15

School and work

The impact of endometriosis on women+'s lives can be profound, and while we 'can no longer afford to ignore it', diagnosis pathways, treatment costs and research investment remain underfunded. In Australia, the five-year NAPE expired in July 2023, with many initiatives that received seed or one-off funding, struggling to continue or finish their work.

A ground-breaking qualitative study involving Australian women+ by Moradi et al. (2014) revealed impacts on study, work, marital/sexual relationships, social and sporting life, and on physical and psychological health. For younger women+ aged 16 to 24, managing symptoms while pursuing study and education was reported to be difficult. Two-thirds of respondents had taken time off and were less productive.

For those aged 25 to 34, life opportunities, employment and career prospects were impacted by endometriosis, with symptoms limiting the type of work they could do; women+ needing to take time off to manage symptoms; and women+ going part time, leaving a great job or losing the opportunity for promotion. As a result of endometriosis, women+ suffer financial loss or a decrease in income due to working part time, not having paid sick leave or having to use leave entitlements for scheduled surgery.

The years of healthy life lost and the impact on those living with endometriosis are measured for economic purposes as a 'non-fatal burden'. In 2023, The Australian Burden of Disease Study estimated that 8213 years of healthy life were lost due to endometriosis in Australia, a rate of 0.61 per 1000 females. The disease burden due to endometriosis is highest among females aged 30 to 34, with a rate of 1.71 years of healthy life lost per 1000 females. This is at a time when women+ are in an aspirational phase of life, with an established career path, possibly romantically partnered, and looking to purchase a property and start a family.

A global, multicentre study of 1418 women+ (aged 18 to 45 years) with endometriosis reported that each woman+ lost an average of 10.8 hours of work weekly because of lower work productivity, mainly owing to reduced effectiveness while working. The study 'demonstrated that pelvic pain and disease severity are the major drivers of work productivity loss in endometriosis. Although reduced effectiveness at work is less frequently assessed and recorded than work absence, it accounted for nearly 60 per cent of total work productivity loss.'

Endo girls

With an average delay in diagnosis of 6.5 years in Australia, young women+ with endo are robbed of their carefree years, instead suffering pain, invalidation, misunderstanding and dismissal. These endo warriors could receive treatment earlier to manage their symptoms, allowing them to participate in life with fewer limitations and to be empowered to take advantage of study and work opportunities.

One-third of 14-year-old girls have serious menstrual pain, according to a 20-year study by Murdoch Children's Research Institute and the University of Melbourne, which involved 1600 adolescents; for girls aged between 16 and 18, around half experienced the same serious pain. The study reports that: 'Thirty-five percent of participants at 14 years of age, 50 per cent at 16 years, and 46 per cent at 18 years reported dysmenorrhea (very or quite painful periods)'.

Due to period pain, overall, the 'quality of life and participation in school, sport, and social activities are all affected. As a result, they were three to five times more likely than those without pain or with "a little" pain to miss school or university.'

A review of recent evidence and guidelines published in 2024 in the *Australian Journal of General Practice* recommends that GPs: 'Refer young people (aged 17 years and under) with suspected or confirmed endometriosis to a paediatric and adolescent gynaecologist with an interest in endometriosis or to a gynaecologist who is comfortable treating adolescents with possible endometriosis.'

It is crucial the awareness of what is 'normal' begins in primary schools, and is cemented in secondary school, with school nurses the conduit to parents, who, in turn, confidently take their daughters to the GP for referral, diagnosis and treatment of their symptoms, especially persistent pelvic pain.

A study by Cameron et al. (2024) found that those with period pain were up to five times more likely to miss school and three times more likely to skip sports than those without it.

In a study of 1835 girls from the Longitudinal Study of Australian Children (LSAC), 1600 (87 per cent) answered questions about their periods. At age 14, 35 per cent reported period pain, which increased to 50 per cent at age 16 and slightly decreased to 46 per cent at age 18. Of the 366 girls who reported their pain across all three age points, 37 per cent never had period pain, 18 per cent had it consistently, 24 per cent reported worsening pain over time, and 10 per cent said their pain lessened.

A significant number of girls missed activities, defined as school, work, social, sport and exercise, due to period pain: 34 per cent at ages 14 and 16, and 31 per cent at age 18. Those with very painful periods were more likely to miss activities, with 72 per cent missing at least one a month at age 14, 63 per cent at age 16, and 65 per cent at age 18.

The study concludes that a large number of adolescent girls in Australia suffer from period pain, which affects their daily activities, including school. Recognising and addressing period pain early is important, not only for improving their quality of life but also for early detection of potential chronic conditions like endometriosis.

Teachers need to step up

At school, period pain is often dismissed as normal, leading to stigma and inadequate treatment. As we've discussed, it involves a complex mix of social, psychological and biological factors. Persistent pelvic pain can harm mental health, and stress can make the pain worse.

Teachers, coaches and school nurses are on the frontline. They see firsthand when their students don't come to school, have trouble concentrating, won't participate in sports, and seek support and medication for pain relief. They have the opportunity and authority to advocate for their students to parents, suggest pathways for diagnosis and raise awareness of what is, and importantly, is not normal.

Persistent pelvic pain, including but not limited to endometriosis, is often overlooked. While endometriosis has gained more attention and funding, we need to invest in educating school staff—teachers, nurses and sports coaches—in recognising and treating period and pelvic pain in adolescents as absolutely necessary to improve their long-term quality of life.

Understanding menstrual health is crucial for developing effective public health education strategies for girls and women+ living with life-defining, lifelong symptoms and impacts of endometriosis and other reproductive health conditions, starting in primary school.

The stigma of the treatments, usually the common OCP, can also have a really detrimental effect on girls when they need to 'hand it over' with medications for school events and camps to teachers or coaches. Discretion, sensitivity and privacy are fundamental in front of other students. Unfortunately, teenagers are cruel and reputational damage about presumed or perceived sexual activity is damaging to girls. I urge school communities to treat their students with compassion and care.

LongSTEPPP

The Longitudinal Study of Teenagers with Endometriosis, Period and Pelvic Pain (LongSTEPPP) is a five-year Australian study that will run from 2022 to 2027. It is led by Professor Sonia Grover and Dr Courtney Munro from the Murdoch Children's Research Institute in Melbourne and supported by children's hospitals across Australia.

The premise for the research is that 'period and pelvic pain can be managed to prevent chronic pain and endometriosis'.

The LongSTEPPP Co-Design Periods Survey was an anonymous online survey conducted as part of a larger five-year project studying periods and pelvic pain in Australian teenagers with endometriosis. The survey aimed to understand adolescents' experiences with menstruation to develop better patient-reported outcome measures.

Adolescents aged 12 to 18 who had been menstruating for at least three months and could consent were invited to participate, mostly through social media. Of the 1811 participants, 85 per cent reported that their periods had a 'moderate' or greater impact on their lives.

Common reasons for missing activities included pain (90.7 per cent), heavy flow (56.2 per cent) and worry about leakage (49 per cent). Menstrual symptoms ranged from cramping and nausea to low energy and mood changes.

The problem of girls missing school because of persistent pelvic pain and painful periods will remain invisible until schools are made to 'track' reasons for absences. When seeking help for their periods, 39.8 per cent of adolescents consulted a general practitioner, 21.3 per cent saw their school nurse and nearly 1 in 10 (9.3 per cent) spoke with a mental health practitioner. To manage their symptoms, most used heat packs (66 per cent), over-the-counter medications (55.8 per cent), and prescription medications (28.6 per cent).

The survey revealed a lack of menstrual health awareness among adolescents, highlighting the significant impact of periods on their lives and the various methods they use to manage symptoms.

Be aware

You can join the LongSTEPPP study, and the pre-screening questionnaire is in the resources. You are eligible to join the study if:
- you are aged 10 to 18 years
- you experience pelvic or period pain and have seen your GP about it or have been referred to a gynaecologist
- you live in Australia
- both you and one of your parents/guardians are willing to take part.

You cannot take part in this study if:
- you're unable to read and understand English
- you can't complete the questionnaires online
- your parent/guardian doesn't want to be involved.

Be prepared

As a part of the study, you will be asked to complete the LongSTEPPP questionnaires once a year for five years. It takes between 30 and 50 minutes to answer all the questions. The questionnaire is online and can be done at your own pace.

In the questionnaire, you and your parent/guardian will be asked questions about periods, pain, quality of life and mental health. Your parent/guardian won't see your answers and you won't see theirs.

School education

The Periods, Pain and Endometriosis Program (PPEP Talk) is an initiative of the Pelvic Pain Foundation of Australia, and funded by the federal Australian Government Department of Health and Aged Care, with support from state and territory governments. PPEP Talk is an Australian program presented across government, Catholic and independent schools.

PPEP Talk is a fun, medically accurate and age-appropriate information session incorporating modern neuroscience research on pain, and is of benefit to all students, particularly the one in four girls and people assigned female at birth with severe period pain. Approximately half of these girls and women+ will develop endometriosis during their teens and twenties. The program lasts one hour and is delivered by fully trained educators. It incorporates animation, video and interactive components. It includes specifically developed resources for use during the session, and resources for girls with pain to take home and discuss with their parents.

This curriculum-linked health and wellbeing education program is aimed at year 10 students when most will have begun menstruating. The 60-minute session is followed by an opportunity for individual students or teachers with specific or personal pain concerns to discuss these with the program educator individually. PPEP Talk provides early intervention and supports girls, families, teachers and schools at a time when pain is more easily managed, and the life effects of pain and missed school can be most efficiently minimised. The clinical educators delivering PPEP Talk have health qualifications and undergo extensive in-house training.

PPEP Talk has also been adapted for intellectual and developmental disabilities, sports, trans and gender diversity, cultural and linguistic diversity, prisons and youth detention, Yarns (the passing on of information and cultural knowledge for Aboriginal and Torres Strait Islanders) and the workplace.

Endo gendernomics

Gendernomics in women+'s health examines how economic principles and gender dynamics intersect to affect women+'s health outcomes, access to care, and overall wellbeing. It highlights the systemic inequalities and biases that women+ face within healthcare systems, emphasising the need for targeted interventions to improve health equity, gender inequality, inclusion and diversity, and the broader economic consequences. This includes narrowing the gender pay gap.

Medical misogyny results from conscious and unconscious bias. The Australian Government National Strategy to Achieve Gender Equality review reports that 'Women disproportionately experience delayed diagnosis, overprescribing, and a failure to properly investigate symptoms'.

So far, you have read examples of entrenched systemic, intersectional and plain sexism girls and women+ face in the general Australian community. This is demonstrably worse for those experiencing the taboos of the 'P Party': periods, painful sex, poo and pee problems.

UTERUSopia: equity for those born with uteruses

In an ideal world, the one in seven women+ diagnosed with a chronic, lifelong disease that periodically (pardon the pun) disrupts their lives would be considered sympathetically, with accommodations made and flexibility available when required.

This culture of sympathy and understanding, without judgement or gender discrimination, would ensure true gender equity by also supporting caregivers when their partner, wife, daughter, mother or sister needs them.

These needs extend to times when they have heavy menstrual bleeding, crippling pain, brain fog, need to attend medical appointments for chronic care, have undergone surgery and are recovering, or are dealing with fertility treatment and pregnancy loss.

UTERUSurper: rights removed from those born with uteruses

If these needs are not met, the women+ living with an already life-defining, incurable disease become more marginalised and underemployed; join the casualised workforce; do not accrue or have any leave entitlements to manage their symptoms and attend medical appointments; can't afford private health insurance; and become so intersectionally disadvantaged they will never fulfil their potential. This lack of fulfilment and economic distress impacts their mental health.

It also costs the economy and the community as a whole through lost productivity, higher social security payments and enormous pressure on the already overburdened public health system. Then there's housing—if these women+ can't work because employers are not accommodating their health needs, they can't afford to pay rent, let alone buy a house.

Their economic security diminishes, but their endometriosis remains a constant unwanted usurper of the life they deserve; it seizes power over their lives, robs them of choice, and too often denies them intimate relationships and children of their own.

Endo's impact on under- and unemployment

Raising awareness about the impact of endometriosis on women+ in the workplace is crucial, as the condition significantly affects both employees and employers across all industries. Endometriosis can lead to debilitating symptoms such as pelvic pain, heavy periods, extreme fatigue, and other chronic issues that can hinder work performance and career progression. Women+ with endometriosis often experience absenteeism (missing work) and presenteeism (being at work but not fully productive).

Reproductive leave is on the gender equity agenda being considered by government unions and employer groups. Despite the name, it isn't really about reproduction or having a baby. It encompasses a range of conditions and treatments, allowing employees time off for issues such as menstruation, menopause, endometriosis, polycystic ovarian syndrome, fertility treatments (including IVF) and procedures like hysterectomies. I prefer 'Women's+ Health leave', adopted by the Australian Financial Complaints Authority (AFCA) in 2023. Female employees are now entitled to five days paid leave to support their unique health needs across all life stages. This includes, but is not limited to, menstruation, fertility care, endometriosis and menopause. This benefit is also available to employees who have female reproductive organs but do not identify as women.

The ombudsman service also increased early pregnancy loss leave from 5 to 10 days paid, per circumstance, while employees or their partner who experience pregnancy loss after the first 20 weeks of pregnancy will now be entitled to take 18 weeks paid leave.

In Australia, reproductive leave is not universally mandated and varies significantly across different workplaces. It is not part of the National Employment Standards, meaning that employees do not automatically have access to it unless their employer provides it through enterprise agreements or workplace policies.

The primary aim of reproductive leave is to provide employees with the necessary time off to manage personal health challenges, without the fear of losing income or job security. The benefits include:

- Support for health management: Employees can take time off for medical appointments, treatments or recovery from conditions that disproportionately affect women+ and other gender-diverse individuals.
- Reduction in stigma: By recognising reproductive health as a legitimate reason for leave, workplaces can foster a more inclusive environment that reduces stigma around these issues.
- Improved workforce retention: Reproductive leave may help retain workers who might otherwise leave due to health-related challenges. This is particularly relevant in sectors with high female representation, such as healthcare and education.
- Economic benefits: This leave allows individuals to manage their health effectively, contributing to closing the gender pay gap and enhancing overall workforce productivity.

Empowering those living with endometriosis and their circle with the knowledge and safe space to discuss managing endometriosis symptoms and time impacts at work promotes flexibility. It improves productivity and retention of great women+ with experience and corporate memory.

A workplace assistance program that aims to support women+ living with the life-impacting symptoms of endometriosis and challenges like fertility and surgical treatment leads to endo empowerment, ultimately improving outputs for staff and their workplaces and the wellbeing of those living with endometriosis or caring for them. The cost of under- or unemployment and casualised jobs impacts the financial security of women+ living with endometriosis, and their ability to pay for treatment and health insurance. According to a report from the Australian Department of Prime Minister and Cabinet 'We could add $128 billion to the economy through boosting women's workforce participation and productivity growth if we tackle the factors holding women back.'

About Bloody Time

In March 2024, 1700 endometriosis sufferers responded to a news .com.au survey titled About Bloody Time, and more than '83 per cent of respondents said they had taken time off work because of their perpetual pain, but more than half admitted they were suffering in secret — choosing not to tell their boss for fear of being disbelieved or even sacked.'

In addition to the impact of living with endo on workplace attendance, the job security and financial hit arising from taking time off work, health costs highlight the 'endo gendernomics' disadvantage.

Respondents shared that medical bills have 'forced' many women+ living with debilitating symptoms to avoid the cost of diagnosis and treatment, leaving them with 'unresolved pain'. Over 50 per cent of respondents report spending over $5000 on their treatment, and 71 respondents $100 000 (About Bloody Time survey outcomes, 2024).

According to the AIHW report on endometriosis, there is no data on the wait for endometriosis surgery in the public system. It estimates that half of patients waited for their procedure for less than three months (within 78 days), with 90 per cent seen within almost a year (354 days).

It reports that most endometriosis-related hospitalisations were partly or fully funded by private health insurance (58 per cent), and only 28 per cent were for public patients, yet over two-thirds (68 per cent) took place in a private hospital.

One in ten women+ 'self-fund' their surgery — they can't wait, being in 'excruciating pain' as per the medical definition for those with stage 4 endometriosis. Therefore, women+ who have surgery for endometriosis may have already been in a better financial position to be able to afford their surgery, and this is an indictment on Australia's so-called 'universal' health system.

If you can't afford private health insurance or to pay your own hospital and specialist costs as a result of endo gendernomics, you will be among the 31.5 per cent relying upon the public health system, at risk of languishing in pain, like 7.7 per cent or the 652 women+ who waited over one year for 'elective' endo surgery in 2021–22. This is simply not acceptable.

Choosing health and happiness: Julie's story

Julie Snook is an endo warrior and a media star on all platforms, including the *Canberra Weekly Magazine,* Southern Cross Austereo, Mix 106.3, and Channel Nine. She resigned from her high-profile media role because of her endo and currently hosts Sky's flagship racing program, Racing Dreams. Julie has endured 13 endometriosis operations since the age of 19. Due to scarring from inflammation and surgeries, a hysterectomy is next on the agenda. Julie supported the news.com.au About Bloody Time campaign to voice concern for those who cannot afford to pay the costs to treat their disease.

> *As a teenager, for years, I had experienced odd bouts of illness. Migraines, severe back and body pain, collapsing at school ... I was just a kid. Despite the many hospital and doctor visits, nothing really came of it.*
>
> *At age 18, I was a fresh-faced cadet journalist working at a regional newspaper, and these symptoms kept intensifying. I remember going back to the same GP at least three times pleading my case, that something wasn't right. Was it IBS, was it migraines, was it in my head? Eventually, I asked for a referral to a gynaecologist. The doctor was almost defensive when I did so—deep down, I don't think she believed me.*
>
> *I travelled the hour to the next major town for my appointment with the specialist. Within minutes of reading my wad of files, he said, 'I think it's endometriosis, but I'll have to operate to know.' Endometry-what-now?*
>
> *Needless to say, I had never heard of this as a teenager growing up in country New South Wales. It wasn't taught to us at school; no GP seemed to know about it.*
>
> *But on this day, the specialist sitting in front of me did know about it, and I had no choice but to trust him. So, I said naively, 'OK, let's operate'. I underwent the surgery a short time later. I took*

one day off work, thinking this procedure would be straightforward and non-invasive. I briefly mentioned it to my mum and didn't bother worrying dad. How naïve I was.

I saw the specialist in the hours after my procedure and he confirmed it was endometriosis that had been plaguing me all this time. But, fingers crossed, he got it all, and the recovery would be hasty.

Over the years, I've hosted red carpets and rolling news coverage, sporting shows and corporate clients. I've witnessed some of the world's greatest moments and some of our hardest too... all in a job that I absolutely loved. All the while I was carrying a chronic condition that has no cure. All the while I was spending thousands of dollars, outside of private health cover, to pay for medical appointments. All the while I was trialling various medications and complementary treatments. Because that is all you can do when you have this condition.

When you're sitting at a news desk or holding a microphone, people can't see the heat pack on your stomach, the heat patches on your back... they don't know makeup is covering the bags from lost sleep, or your handbag doubling as a small pharmacy to help you when the symptoms unexpectedly arise.

I don't want to make this political, but what I do want is for all those suffering... to have access to appropriate and affordable healthcare services. It shouldn't be a choice.

In 2019, I did make a choice. I chose to step away from my dream job in a national newsroom, and I chose my health and my future. I married the love of my life and stepped away from stressful, often confronting work as a journalist. Instead, I prioritised projects I'm passionate about, health and happiness.

Not every patient is that fortunate... there are countless instances of females forced to choose a hysterectomy over monthly agony... couples forced to choose whether their hearts, and bank accounts, can endure another round of IVF... individuals forced to choose to let go of finding a partner because dating with endo is 'too hard'.

Endometriosis is often referred to as a silent disease because we can't see it, but its implications are deafening.

On the 16th of December 2022, my driving force through all of the pain ... was placed in my arms for the first time, weighing 8 pounds and 3 ounces.

That little boy changed my life in that one moment ... and made all the years prior worth it. My son is my reason to celebrate.

To the million women living with this condition, learning of this condition, just trying with this condition, you are not alone, it is not in your head and you will get through.

Endometriosis and the workplace

The impact of endometriosis is estimated to cost the Australian economy $9.7 billion annually through lost productivity and healthcare costs. This underscores the need for employers to support workers with endometriosis and make reasonable adjustments to help them perform their jobs effectively.

Recent research from Bourdon et al. in 2024 involving 1557 French women+ found that endometriosis harms the professional wellbeing of 65 per cent of women+, and 62 per cent declare they are physically and intellectually impaired by symptoms.

Endometriosis and workplace expectations can be managed together, increasing productivity and safeguarding 'corporate memory'. Finding well-qualified employees is difficult, and endo warriors are the type of resilient employee in demand.

What does the research tell us

Professor Gita Mishra's team at the University of Queensland's Women's Health Australia found that women+ who had surgery for endometriosis were 85 per cent more likely to be unemployed three years after their diagnosis than before, and that 63 per cent of women+ born in 1973–78 who had surgery for endometriosis were working fulltime before diagnosis, a number that dropped to 44 per cent after their diagnosis.

A large study in Switzerland, Germany and Australia (Does endometriosis affect professional life?) found that women+ with endometriosis had to consider health-related limitations in their career decisions to a significantly higher degree than women+ in the control group, that chronic pain was significantly associated with increased sick leave as well as with loss of productivity at work, and that women+ with endometriosis were less often able to work in their desired profession than women+ without endometriosis.

Of those diagnosed with endometriosis, 89.8 per cent noted a loss of work productivity due to endometriosis, with 65.1 per cent reporting strong or very strong limitations when symptoms were severe. Even on days when they weren't having strong endometriosis symptoms, 75.3 per cent still felt some degree of loss of productivity.

They reported that 13.1 per cent had used one week or more of overtime or vacation during the previous year when they felt too sick to work due to symptoms of endometriosis. During the previous month, 75.5 per cent of women+ with endometriosis reported having gone to work despite severe pain, and 89.2 per cent of women+ confirmed that they had worked in the previous year regardless of pain.

Among those with endometriosis, 10.3 per cent reported working parttime, with 5.8 per cent stopping work completely due to their disease and symptoms. Flexibility and a sympathetic workplace culture is urgently needed. With the proper support, employees with endometriosis can continue to thrive in their careers.

Who's responsible for workplace health and safety?

Safe Work Australia is responsible for the national policy for workplace health and safety. The Commonwealth, states and territories regulate and enforce workplace health and safety laws.

The Fair Work Ombudsman provides education, assistance, advice and guidance to employers, employees and organisations. It promotes and monitors compliance with workplace laws, enquires into and investigates breaches of the *Fair Work Act* 2009, and takes appropriate enforcement action.

Be mindful that, under the *Work Health and Safety Act* (Section 28), workers must take reasonable care of their own psychological and physical health and safety, and not adversely affect the health and safety of other persons. They must comply with reasonable health and safety instructions, as far as they are reasonably able, and cooperate with reasonable health and safety policies or procedures.

Suppose you're in a job that requires your attention, and you are responsible for others. In that case, it is important to understand that, while employers have fair work, occupational health and safety obligations, so do you as an employee. For example, WorkSafe Victoria advises: 'While at work, workers must take reasonable care for their health and safety, and that others may be affected by the worker's acts or omissions.'

So, when you're really struggling with symptoms, please speak to your line manager or other work colleagues about how you're affected and take care of yourself and those around you. Communication and accommodation are key to protecting yourself and your colleagues.

Endometriosis is an invisible disease, and your colleagues might only notice occasional flare-ups; let's face it, most workmates will be oblivious to your symptoms, and the stigma around the 'P party' symptoms makes them—and you—uncomfortable talking about it. To raise awareness of your health needs and support, which can help you maintain your employment, you need to disclose and discuss your challenges. This is not easy; advocating for yourself while opening up about personal symptoms can feel embarrassing.

A recent study by the University of Melbourne researchers Ghin et al. found that even though leaders struggle with discussing chronic health conditions, almost three-quarters deliberately hide their chronic illness at work. If your boss isn't being honest about their own health challenges, how can you feel safe discussing your own?

Training managers about endometriosis is the missing piece in the puzzle. They need to trust you, respect you and understand that you're not seeking an advantage; you simply need a level playing field to help you achieve the business goals and meet your key performance indicators. It is up to them to manage the workplace policies, set criteria and ensure adjustments and flexibility don't become a 'free for all', creating a precedent for other colleagues to take advantage.

Employee rights and workplace flexibility in Australia

In Australia, the *Fair Work Act* 2009 provides a framework for employee rights, workplace health and safety, and flexibility in work arrangements. Here's an overview of how these elements interact to support employees.

The *Fair Work Act* ensures that all employees have specific rights and protections, including:

- General protections: Employees are entitled to protection against unlawful discrimination, adverse actions and coercion in the workplace. This includes protections related to race, gender, disability and other personal characteristics, such as a chronic health condition.
- Right to flexible work arrangements: Employees may request flexible work arrangements if they meet certain criteria, such as being a parent or caregiver or if they have a disability. Employers are required to consider these requests seriously and can only refuse on reasonable business grounds.
- Occupational health and safety: The *Act* mandates that employers provide a safe workplace, which includes addressing health issues that may affect employees, including chronic conditions like endometriosis. Employers must take reasonable steps to ensure the health and safety of their employees.

Balancing workplace commitments: Kristina's story

Kristina Luburic is the managing director of Global VML Health in Australia and New Zealand. Kristina is an experienced healthcare communication specialist with a career spanning over 20 years in the pharmaceutical marketing industry. She has worked across multiple areas, including oncology, cardiology, respiratory, endocrinology, psychiatry and ophthalmology, and has a personal interest in endometriosis.

'As soon as I started to get my periods at the age of 12, I realised my friends' experience wasn't as severe as mine.' Kristina wasn't taken seriously, and her pain was dismissed for years.

I think in my early uni days, I knew that my symptoms were getting worse, but I wasn't ever diagnosed. I had mentioned to doctors that I had severe period pain, and they told me, 'That's just what happens; some people have more or less period pain'.

School and work **217**

Kristina soldiered on like a good endo warrior despite the pain and was in her late 20s when she got answers.

I ended up having to do emergency surgery because I had a cyst on my ovary that was the size of an orange. They also found many endometriosis lesions during the laparoscopy as well, and the scarring was so severe that there were parts of it that just couldn't be removed.

This diagnosis was a validating moment for her as it confirmed that her pain was not imagined, and she had another two laparoscopies. 'Both times, it was due to chocolate cysts, and they were both emergency surgeries.'

Kristina remembers the impact of 'really heavy menstrual bleeding'.

Growing up, I was raised in a very low socioeconomic family, and...we couldn't afford pads, so my mum would get old bed sheets. She would rip them up and fold them up, and that would be the pads that I used, but because my bleeding was so heavy, it would just seep through.

She was in such 'significant pain to the point where you're just curled up on the floor, and you cannot move' and so very often incapacitated. She highlights the anxiety of managing endometriosis symptoms alongside academic and professional responsibilities.

When you start into the world of employment, your salary depends on you physically being there; other people physically rely on you being there. There were so many times that, as much as I tried to always be at work, sometimes it was just physically impossible. My employer could probably map monthly when I had to take my 'period' leave until I got to the point where I ran out of sick leave.

Kristina reflects on the lack of support and understanding she experienced for decades, and emphasises the importance of a supportive and empathetic work environment and organisational change.

I think back to when I was younger, there was a really strong stigma. So, it was something that you would never discuss with an employer, particularly a male employer, heaven forbid... But I do feel that now things have shifted. We talk about endometriosis within the business and from a leadership perspective, and we support people throughout their health journey.

I think that's imperative from a leadership perspective and from a management perspective, and organisational change is required to ensure that people feel safe, that they're in an open environment where they can have these conversations, and that people won't judge them negatively.

She urges women+ to 'have a voice and, if they do speak up, they should expect real empathy in a workplace environment'.

Kristina has tried various treatments, including acupuncture and physiotherapy, but highlights the financial burden of managing a lifelong condition. She stresses the need for increased government investment in endometriosis awareness, treatment advancements and equality in healthcare access. 'I hope that the government recognises this need, and they put their money where their mouth is, and they do support women+ with endometriosis and related diseases.'

Having endo in the corporate environment: Antara's story

Antara Mascarenhas has had a distinguished business career in senior marketing and management roles in the energy and climate sector. She is now a policy leader fellow at the European University Institute in Florence, Italy. Her journey with endometriosis has been parallel to her career, and coming from a non-Anglo diverse background has added intersectionality as a challenge.

Her message is about seeking medical help early and openly communicating in the workplace.

My philosophy has always been that they can hear about my endometriosis if I have to deal with it. That's the least they can do. But it isn't easy when you have a professional working relationship. I hope this won't even be an issue when we get to the next generation.

For those reading this, I say be confident that the struggle you've been through with endometriosis makes you a stronger person. You can apply that to whatever you're doing in your life and career and contribute as much or more as the next person because you've gained that resilience of something that you've dealt with relatively young in your life, either as a teenager or probably in your early 20s. And that's a difficult time. Know that you're coming from a place of strength.

My painful symptoms started when I was 12. Every three or four months, I would have an excruciating period. I'd wake up in the morning early with pain and a kind of nausea; I would be on the verge of fainting. I'd go back to sleep after taking some pain medication.

I moved to Canberra from Melbourne, and that's essential context because I was away from my family. I was in a new city. I was around new people. I didn't know anyone, and it was my first week of work as a policy graduate when I felt a bit of pain on the last day of the first week.

I went across the road to do an errand, came back and, very suddenly, I had extreme pain. I started getting sweaty and nauseous, and I fainted right there in the middle of my work pod. The next thing I knew, I opened my eyes, and the graduate coordinator was standing above me, and they had called an ambulance. So that wasn't the entry I wanted to make into the new workplace. As I was put into the ambulance, I could see my GM [general manager] because they'd all come to see what was wrong and help. And I remember feeling mortified.

When I arrived at Canberra Hospital, the doctor never mentioned endometriosis. No-one mentioned it. They put me on a drip. I got my strength back and I was discharged later that day. Fortunately, my supervisor at work suggested a very good GP who referred me to a specialist. I was lucky to land on my feet there. The gynaecologist suggested it could be endometriosis and that I have a laparoscopy. I decided not to take her advice.

Being 25, I figured I could probably live through the pain. I didn't want to spend two grand on an operation when I could use it on travel or save money. In hindsight, this wasn't the best decision. The sooner I had been diagnosed, the sooner I could have treated it. But I think that speaks to the expense involved in diagnosing endo. At that point in my life, I just wanted to be like my peers — go out on Friday night and have fun because I was 25 and living in a new city. I didn't want to deal with it, and I didn't.

I ended up needing to tell my boss each time we did rotations because, once a month, I would wake up in extreme pain and need to manage it with Panadeine Forte. I would be late into the office. My manager was very understanding; he'd raised two daughters on his own.

I foolishly proceeded on for a couple of years, living with the pain until it got to the point where the pain was just so extreme that I fainted every month. Finally, I found an oral contraceptive pill ... that reduced the pain, and the level of bleeding decreased significantly. I kept going with that until I had the laparoscopy, which was about six years later.

No-one had ever discussed fertility with me. I wasn't concerned about it. The most significant issues were pain and heavy menstrual bleeding.

After the laparoscopy, the pain reduced when they removed the endo, and I also had some adhesions. But the bleeding was just very, very heavy. I have memories of travelling when the bleeding was so heavy I couldn't go anywhere; I had to be stuck in the apartment, back and forth to the bathroom.

Being in the office is challenging as well. It makes you weak when you're losing blood. Recently, I've started taking some medication for something unrelated to endometriosis, and that has increased the pain. As a result, I'm now back in that space where I need to be planning ahead, understanding where I will be on the day that I get my period, so I'm not caught out.

School and work   **221**

I mentioned endometriosis to HR in a previous organisation and asked, 'Do you think it would be worth training managers to understand endometriosis and other chronic health conditions?' They said we should leave that to the managers to research.

The workplace culture has changed significantly in the last few years. COVID has been a game changer in that way. It's put chronic health conditions on the map.

I think the diversity of voices now has also changed. There are more women in senior roles. People of diverse backgrounds are now given opportunities that they weren't a few years ago. When I was first a GM, I was one of two females out of about 22 GMs and the only one not Anglo-Saxon or of European background. You can imagine that it wasn't an easy kind of culture working in a pretty, male-dominated industry to [be able to] influence others.

Awareness is growing, and endometriosis is discussed much more in the media — that's really positive. More people have heard of and learnt about endometriosis and its impacts.

Early in my career, it was hard to talk about these things because people perceived women's health, bleeding and period pain as weaknesses. They perceive it as something that's going to affect productivity. I think there is still a way to go regarding culture change to provide the environment for people to talk to their managers about endo and other conditions. As I gained seniority, discussing endometriosis didn't bother me because I had proven myself, backed by my record.

Flexibility, having that opportunity to be in the office and at home when needed, enables many more people to contribute... Working from home isn't a foreign concept now, following the pandemic. I hope we can build a culture where women living with endometriosis can be open about it, seek support when they need it and have open communication with empathy so that people aren't scared to raise it.

I've certainly found, not just at work but in my life, that men are a bit uncomfortable when you talk about your periods. If HR departments speak about menstruation, normalising it, then there doesn't have to be this awkwardness when you have to tell a male boss about your endometriosis. It shouldn't be awkward.

If you don't have endo, it's good on you to listen to this because you are taking the time to educate yourself and be sympathetic to others. If you're a man, even better! We need you to understand and educate yourselves to support us. I was lucky my dad had so much empathy. When I was in pain as a teenager, he would be the one helping me find the pain medication, or if I was out of pads, he'd run to the chemist and get them for me.

Be understanding, be kind, be informed and be endometriosis aware.

Australian workplace law

Before talking to your line manager, employer or business owner, educate yourself about the workplace policies in place, who's who in the human resources zoo, the process and any applications needed to seek support. These may be called grievances (unfair treatment) or complaints policies. Don't feel intimidated; these are terms used for employee and employer communication processes.

It is important to document all interactions with your employer and with all staff relating to your request for workplace support to manage endometriosis. This protects you if they don't fulfil their obligations to you as an employee with a medical condition as required by law. You should record any instances you are discriminated against because of your health issues, directly (if you are overlooked for a promotion, pay rise or higher duties) or indirectly (if you can't comply with a rule or workplace policy because of your medical condition).

Australian workplace laws require employers to make 'reasonable adjustments' to help you do your job. However, they have the right to argue that accommodating your needs will cause hardship for the business or stop you from doing essential parts of the role you were hired to do.

As an accredited workplace mediator, I encourage an impartial, structured information-sharing process and honest disclosures. The mediation process is useful; relationships can be preserved and strengthened, allowing the expression of feelings and psychological, social and economic dynamics relating to you and your work.

Mediation assists the employee and the employer to understand their own and each other's perspectives, issues, motivations and intentions, facilitating conversations and genuine participation in the process.

Don't be alarmed if your employer uses the term 'dispute resolution'. This is a legal term under the *Fair Work Act* (2019), and it includes mediation (an informal process), conciliation (a semi-formal discussion between you and your employer) and arbitration (a formal process with evidence, arguments and a Fair Work Commission decision).

You can also ask for a support person to be present when you meet with your employer. However, they are not obligated to allow this, even if discussions are around possible dismissal (*Fair Work Act 2009* s.387(d)). If you can have a support person, it is a requirement that they 'do not act as an advocate—a support person does not present or defend a case on behalf of the employee'.

The art of asking

Write down a couple of paragraphs about your 'ask'. For example, 'I have endometriosis. Here's some information about how this incurable, chronic disease impacts me. You can learn more at EndoZone (endozone.com.au). To be my best self and most productive, this is the support I need from you at work. When I have flare-ups, medical appointments and new treatments, we need a contingency plan. What can we do to foster open communication and reduce stigma in our workplace?'

Some of the accommodations that you might want to talk to your manager about include:

- taking regular 20-minute rest breaks to help you manage symptoms
- pacing tasks to prevent burnout
- reducing your workload and planning around flare-ups or monthly cycles
- modifying your work tasks to help you manage your pain
- minimising exposure to high-stress situations
- adjusting the work area—for instance, controlling noise or adjusting lighting and temperature
- working from home if recommended by the treating doctor.

Be prepared

You can help facilitate the process of educating your workplace about your condition and managing your needs day to day. Here are a few tips:

- Understand how your symptoms affect your work so you are better able to communicate them.
- Gather information so you can explain your condition and your needs confidently.
- Choose the right time (e.g. not when there is a looming deadline or busy period).
- Find a quiet, private space (such as an office or meeting room) for an uninterrupted conversation.
- Be honest and direct. Clearly state your diagnosis and its impact on your work.
- Help your manager understand the seriousness of the situation (explain your symptoms and how they affect your health).
- Explain how it affects your work (share specific examples of how your symptoms affect your productivity).
- Contextualise why accommodations are necessary and suggest specific accommodations (such as flexible working hours or remote work during flare-ups).
- Reassure your manager you're not leaving them in the lurch and emphasise your dedication to your work.
- Address any concerns about productivity (and how the requested accommodations will help you meet expectations).
- Practise active listening (be present in the moment and attentive to both verbal and non-verbal cues).
- Be open to feedback and discuss solutions collaboratively.
- Schedule a follow-up meeting to assess how effective the accommodations are.

Remember, advocating for your wellbeing is crucial.

Employer obligations

In Australia, employers have specific obligations under workplace health and safety laws and anti-discrimination legislation to support employees living with the disabling impacts of endometriosis.

- Definition of disability: According to the Safe Work Australia advice, 'Severe endometriosis can also amount to a physical disability' under the *Disability Discrimination Act 1992* (Cth) as it significantly affects a person's ability to carry out normal daily activities.
- Employers are prohibited from discriminating against employees with endometriosis because of their disability. This includes areas such as recruitment, employment terms, promotions, training and dismissals.
- Reasonable adjustments: Employers have a duty to make reasonable adjustments to accommodate employees with endometriosis. These adjustments may involve modifying work arrangements, providing flexible hours, allowing medical appointments or breaks, offering ergonomic equipment or adjusting the physical workplace to meet individual needs.
- Consultation and communication: Employers should communicate openly with employees to understand their condition and its impact on work.
- Confidentiality: Employers must ensure the confidentiality of an employee's medical information, disclosing it only to relevant individuals on a need-to-know basis.
- Discrimination complaints: If an employee believes they've faced discrimination due to endometriosis, they can lodge a complaint. Employers should have internal procedures to address and resolve such issues promptly.

When discussing adjustments with your manager, consider factors such as how the condition affects you, your absence levels, how it might impact the business, and what the potential changes that could help you might be (e.g. modified duties, reduced hours, working from home, and any special equipment).

You will find more information on my website (advisorygovcorp .com.au) on endo-friendly workplaces, mediation and support.

The need for a sympathetic workplace: Kaila's story

Kaila Murnain is an associate partner in communications with global advocacy company SEC Newgate. Prior to this, she was the first and only female general secretary of the New South Wales Labor Party and is a member of the World Economic Forum Global Forum of Young Leaders, an accelerator for a dynamic community of exceptional people with the vision, courage and influence to drive positive change in the world. Kaila holds a Bachelor of Social Science, and Psychological Science (Honours).

She is also an endo warrior who has been living with excruciating pelvic pain, heavy menstrual bleeding, fatigue, digestive issues and difficulty sleeping since she was 17.

I saw more than a dozen doctors and had as many hospitalisations over the years, and endometriosis wasn't mentioned. I learnt about it through a friend, not a medical professional. Like so many women's health problems, it gets brushed away. I was told it could be IBS.

Having symptoms as I did through my teenage years and 20s certainly changed my life choices, particularly things like participating in sports. I love swimming, and it just became more and more difficult. I wish I had been more educated about endometriosis, and I wish I had advocated for myself in a stronger voice. These symptoms make you feel embarrassed and vulnerable. I didn't understand my role in the process. I had to advocate for myself.

I wasn't diagnosed until my late 20s. My symptoms were just normalised, believing that I was perpetually in pain with something that women had to deal with. By the time I started investigating what was going on with me, I'd learnt how to minimise my expression of the pain.

Women didn't discuss the vulnerabilities of heavy menstrual bleeding, pain and certainly not endometriosis. I think that it's changing now with more women in leadership positions generally. In parliament, in councils and, most importantly, in workplaces, we need to support women going through these issues. We have a communal voice, that collegiate voice around women's health issues now that has been building.

I was finally referred to a gynaecologist for treatment. In the end, I had laparoscopic surgery and was found to have stage 4 endometriosis. I had the surgery while I was general secretary of the Labor Party.

The delayed diagnosis could have cost me the opportunity to be a mother, and I feel so blessed to have Ella as my daughter. I wish someone had had a conversation with me about fertility earlier. I was told that the best time to try to conceive was six months after the laparoscopic surgery, but I was in a really important job at the time and put it off. I also didn't realise that fertility treatment is painful. The hormones they use to harvest eggs make you really unwell.

My advice to young girls and women of all ages is that painful periods are not normal. Heavy menstrual bleeding is not just something to put up with. It shouldn't be normalised. We need to support girls and women with these symptoms. Awareness and education are key; with that knowledge, people will have the capacity to advocate for themselves and get the help and support they need with the medical community's commitment.

I'm very pleased to see such non-partisan support for endometriosis, particularly in politics. It's been really important having politicians like Nicolle Flint and Annastacia Palaszczuk, Jacinta Allan and Rachel Payne speak of their own experiences. Strong women build walls around themselves.

We need to have sympathetic workplaces [because] so many women, many of whom are working part time, are in lower-paid jobs because of the challenges associated with their symptoms. I do believe that workplace understanding and respect are fundamental. I'm very pleased to say that my current workplace is fantastic. It is a great place to work.

We have a long, long way to go to ensure workplaces across the country have support for all employees to safeguard the economic security of women and also their mental health. It's a burden enough to carry around a chronic disease, excruciating pain and heavy bleeding. We don't want to increase the burden by making them feel inadequate or unable to speak up about the impact of their symptoms for fear of losing their job. Too many resign from their employment to have endometriosis surgery, recovery and fertility treatment or simply because they don't get the support they need. That's a loss to the employer, the woman and Australia in terms of productivity. We need to do better.

CHAPTER 16
Medical misogyny

I have been a committed and vocal advocate for gender equality, notably raising women+'s rights in my inaugural speech to Parliament when I was elected aged 28, and throughout my career. I chose to deepen my academic understanding of gender, diversity and inclusion impacts in the workplace by completing my Master of Leadership, considering theories, concepts and issues to improve opportunities for girls and women+. Decades of working in politics and the building sector have confirmed we have a long way to go to address gender inequality and sexism.

These fundamental factors also contribute to Australia's women+'s health gap and globally. With intersectionality (when issues of sexism, racism, classism, ageism, ableism, and heterosexism are experienced), the disparities in health outcomes become even more pronounced.

Women+ often face systemic barriers to healthcare access due to entrenched gender norms that prioritise male health needs. Research indicates that women+ are less likely than men to receive necessary medical treatment and financial aid for healthcare costs. For instance, women+ in various communities across many nations report under-utilisation of healthcare services, which can be attributed to traditional gender roles that limit their decision making power regarding health.

How the medical world excludes and ignores women+

In December 2023, the National Women's Health Advisory Council was called to examine medical misogyny. The review is chaired by the Assistant Minister for Health and Aged Care, the Hon. Ged Kearney, who said:

> *Women and girls deserve tailored and targeted healthcare that recognises and reflects their experiences and concerns. Social prejudice, ingrained bias in medical practice and exclusion from research trials and other studies culminate in a medical catastrophe for women… (it is a) combination of social prejudice, ingrained bias in medical practice and exclusion from research trials and other studies culminate in a medical catastrophe for women.*

And medical misogyny extends to testing as well. Until the 1990s, women+ were routinely excluded from drug trials. So medicines to treat women+'s conditions didn't take into account hormones and reproductive realities or the female body — even doses were decided based on men's physiology. Professor Robyn Norton AO from the University of New South Wales notes that 'male-centric' healthcare approaches delay diagnosis and treatment due to knowledge gaps.

A 2019 study of data from the entire Danish population by the Novo Nordisk Foundation Center for Protein Research found that, on average, women+ were diagnosed four years later than men across 770 diseases studied.

On page 69, we talked about the impact of hormone treatments that induce menopause, including lowering bone mineral density. Indeed, the TGA recommends that women+ using these therapies have DEXA bone scans to reduce the risk of osteoporosis.

The Medicare Benefits Schedule item 12312 is used for hypogonadism, when a woman+'s ovaries aren't producing enough estrogen or a man's testes aren't producing enough testosterone. Guess what?! A bloke who has low testosterone has no age restrictions and gets the Medicare rebate in full, no questions asked. Meanwhile, women+, who account for 82 per cent of diagnostic services under this item number, must have had the condition for six months and be under 45 years of age.

Another fun fact is that scrotal (balls) ultrasounds get a higher rebate than female pelvic ultrasounds, which I argue are more complex and take longer.

These are a few examples of discrimination against women+ in favour of men in the medical imaging system. Even women+ without endometriosis are likely to need several ultrasounds and MRIs in their lifetime for 'reproductive', gynaecological and sexual health, and they pay more for a system designed for Adam, not Eve. For those with endometriosis, these tests actively reduce diagnostic delay so treatment and management can be commenced.

End Gender Bias survey

The findings of the Australian-first #EndGenderBias survey released in the endometriosis awareness month of March 2024 revealed that two out of three women+ in Australia experience discrimination in healthcare settings. Common issues include having their pain dismissed or being labelled as 'hysterical' when seeking treatment for serious conditions. This bias leads to delayed diagnoses and inadequate care, particularly for conditions like endometriosis and PCOS where women+'s symptoms are often trivialised.

The 'Minister for Endo', Hon. Ged Kearney MP, Assistant Minister for Health, has been a vocal advocate for more awareness of women+'s health issues.

For too long, women have been suffering unnecessarily. They've been dismissed, ignored and called hysterical. It is unacceptable that two-thirds of women experience bias and discrimination in Australia's health system. It's time we acted on this.

The results of the #EndGenderBias survey are shocking, but not surprising. The report also showed that Australian women+ regularly feel unheard and not taken seriously by their medical practitioners.

The report also found that:

- sexual and reproductive health and chronic pain are the top areas where women+ experience gender bias
- more than 70 per cent of women+ experience bias in the diagnosis and treatment of health conditions
- more than 70 per cent of women+ experience bias during GP visits.

For example, awareness of endometriosis symptoms among younger girls and women+ has grown exponentially, reflected in the rate of hospitalisations, which has doubled among women+ aged 20 to 24 over the past decade.

However, the systemic bias in the Australian health and hospital systems is an indictment on our so-called 'universal' health system. Simply put, 14 per cent of girls and women+ are victims of inequity in a medical system designed by men, for men. This is, thankfully, changing.

The #EndGenderBias Survey Summary reported that women+ have positive experiences when healthcare professionals invest time in discussing options, carefully explaining procedures and asking questions that are sensitive to the woman+'s experience. Women+ want healthcare professionals to be honest about what they don't know, to be open to learning about their individual circumstances, and to acknowledge and explicitly address power imbalances. We know these behaviours are foundational to culturally safe care and trauma-informed care, but they're difficult to achieve in contexts of short consultations, fragmented care and rushed healthcare professionals. Women+ are finding that health professionals who listen — and take their concerns seriously — are often a turning point in women+'s treatment, care and recovery.

The federal government announced a funding package, 'Reforming the health system to improve sexual and reproductive care', which established a gender audit to examine the Medicare rebates for some treatments in women+'s health, such as imaging (e.g. ultrasounds). It is also inquiring into rebates for the insertion and removal of long-acting reversible contraceptives (LARCs) and IUDs, including the Mirena used for endometriosis and adenomyosis. The current rebates aren't enough to cover the costs of the procedure, and doctors argue that, as a result, they and their patients are out of pocket. The 2024 federal budget allocated $5.2 million for scholarships to train healthcare professionals in removing and inserting LARCs for contraception and other medical treatments.

Fighting systemic medical misogyny: Ged's story

The Hon. Ged Kearney is a vocal advocate for women+'s rights when it comes to their health and equitable access to care. She is very open about her 'mission' to tackle medical misogyny.

When I speak about medical misogyny, I feel like I am putting my shoulder against a big mountain. I am trying to shift it because it has so many roots steeped in history, and it is a cultural problem, an economic problem and a gendered problem, of course. We really need to change it from the roots up, and it's proving quite difficult. Nevertheless, I am absolutely determined. I chair the National Women's Health Advisory Council, a wonderful group of health professionals, consumers, academics, researchers and people who understand the problem and want to change it.

When I first raised medical misogyny in parliament and in this role that I'm in now as assistant minister, I was amazed at the number of people who said to me, 'Hey, yay, hallelujah, we've been battling against these things for so long', but there has never been a really coordinated, all-of-government approach to garner all that knowledge, that strength of people, including physicians and women generally who have experienced what I call gender bias or medical misogyny and just really turn the ship around.

I think we really need to empower women. We need to ensure that they are safe in the health system, that their access is equal, and that their outcomes are equal to men's, if not better, certainly better than they are now. We know that outcomes for women in the health system are not as good as men's. And we need to ensure that there is well-funded research to actually enable this to happen.

I learnt about the issues for women who have endometriosis, being gaslit, with medical practitioners telling them that it's just a woman's lot to put up with pain, bad luck, you're drug shopping, you're a little bit hysterical, you're a bit anxious. All of those things

Medical misogyny **235**

that, you know, go with the presentation of a woman when she has pelvic pain. That infuriated me.

[Women are] half as likely to be properly medicated for pain relief, and 78 per cent of people with an autoimmune disease are women, 90 per cent of people who suffer migraines are women. When we did the #EndGenderBias survey, two-thirds of women who responded to that survey said they were discriminated against, dismissed, felt humiliated by the medical system.

This is extraordinary. I was blown away by the depth of women's experiences regarding bias in the health system, and I want to change it. A lot of it's rooted in social prejudice, and it's ingrained in the medical profession. Now, going back a long time, I see that women's health was such a small part of what they learnt. Gynaecologists hardly had endometriosis or pelvic pain in their curriculum, which I find utterly extraordinary.

Over the past two years, I have been travelling around the country listening to women about their experiences in the health system. And what I have learnt is that: Every. Single. Woman. Has a story. From the Kimberley to Melbourne's outer suburbs. From women in the NT to inner city Adelaide.

Every woman has a story about gender bias. About being dismissed or having their symptoms minimised. About an experience of medical misogyny. There are heartbreaking tales of continued pain, of ongoing suffering, of women's long journeys to diagnosis.

As a mother myself, the stories women have told me about care failures around birth trauma are confronting and visceral.

It's outrageous to hear—again and again, we have logged thousands of these stories—that at the most difficult times in their lives, so many women have had to fight to get the care and support they deserve. Not because they were without symptoms or pain or struggle. But because they were women.

I am committed to making change.

GP gender pay gap

The RACGP's 2023 'Health of the Nation Report' noted that 61 per cent of GPs in training were women+. The RACGP also found that women+ GPs in the workforce are more likely to do longer consultations with patients than their male counterparts. Hooray!

I don't know about you, but after spending three minutes finding my notes in the depths of my handbag, going through the sociable 'hellos', as you do, taking a breath to frame our response to the lovely doctor's, 'What can I help you with today?', which prompts a complete mental block, only to realise the notes I'm clutching is the shopping list ... so you dive back into the handbag while making small talk, before finding a 'clean' spot to put your bag down. Time's up.

All the while, the lovely female GP smiles patiently while realising that she's about to be unfairly penalised for spending more time with you than her male counterpart would, meaning she gets a much lower Medicare subsidy for 'lingering longer'. Female GPs are also victims of the gender pay gap.

Bias in research funding

According to the *Closing the Women's Health Gap* report from McKinsey in 2024, despite an estimated 190 million women+ living with endometriosis, 'the market potential for endometriosis treatments is estimated at $180–220 billion globally based on today's share of endometriosis patients seeking treatment. Innovation in this space, including faster diagnosis rates and earlier access to treatment, could increase the market potential'.

Further analysis highlighted in the report for 2019-2023 shows that investment in male erectile dysfunction was USD $1.24 billion, a staggering six times higher than that for endometriosis, which received funding of USD $44 million.

This lack of investment is global. According to UK figures, despite premenstrual syndrome affecting 90 per cent of women+, with serious issues like premenstrual dysphoric disorder (PMDD), there is five times more research into erectile dysfunction, which affects just 19 per cent of men.

Medical and scientific research into endometriosis aims to improve diagnosis, treatment and quality of life. In Australia, the NHMRC's investment in endometriosis research, totalling $18.9 million between 2000 and 2022, and the Medical Research Future Fund's 11 grants since 2015 are insufficient when compared with funding for diseases with similar prevalence. For example, diabetes research funding is significantly higher despite its similar prevalence, affecting approximately one in ten Australians. Over the years, diabetes research has consistently received substantial funding, with competitive grants often exceeding $50 million annually from NHMRC alone.

In the same period, when $29 million was invested in endometriosis by another fund, $530 million was spent on diabetes. This is typical across the international landscape. According to Emma Cox, chief executive of Endometriosis UK, the National Institute for Health Research has funded more than 8000 projects since its inception in 2006, of which, only 11 address endometriosis.

Of course, medical research across all diseases and health conditions is crucial. Just in the time it has taken me to write this book, my immediate family and closest friends have been challenged by diabetes, prostate cancer, leukaemia and heart issues, in addition to hormone, autoimmune and inflammatory conditions.

On balance, funding for medical and scientific research into endometriosis aimed at improving diagnosis, treatment and quality of life has increased since NAPE. However, endometriosis research is underfunded relative to other diseases with high healthcare burdens, possibly due to its complexity and the fact that it only affects women+.

CHAPTER 17

Intersectionality and inclusion in care

Discrimination and marginalisation result in inequality and exclusion of individuals in the health system and throughout society. In this book, we refer to all people born with a uterus for inclusivity as women+, and we have aimed to focus on the person and not the 'difference'.

Intersectional attributes are the different aspects of your identity, relationships and social characteristics. For many women+, gender discrimination is compounded because of their cultural and religious background, gender identity and sexual orientation. For those in geographically isolated and lower socioeconomic circumstances, intersectionality compounds disadvantage.

We will explore the issues faced by diverse groups of people in recognising symptoms of endometriosis, culturally appropriate diagnosis and strategies to navigate the health system.

Culture includes a person's beliefs, and this has a fundamental impact on body image and awareness. A lack of menstrual literacy too often deters women+ from seeking help or treatment.

For many women+, menstruation is taboo, with social or religious customs restricting or forbidding discussion of periods, poo, pee and painful sex, even with other women+. This limits the opportunity for awareness about what is normal and, therefore, the diagnosis and treatment pathways.

Collectively, we need to empower those living with symptoms to advocate for themselves, influence their own health journey and feel heard, understood, supported and, importantly, validated.

The lack of research in this area means that already marginalised communities are further understudied. An integrative and multidisciplinary approach to care is optimal in producing an understanding of the impact of endometriosis. This can only be achieved via open communication that ensures *all* people are heard.

Aboriginal and Torres Strait Islanders

First Nations women+ live with the burden of many diseases compared with other Australian females. Contributing factors include the postcode lottery; living in regional, rural and remote areas; and the cultural norms traditionally held.

Aboriginal and Torres Strait Islander people have a holistic view of health, linked to their own family but extending to the whole community. However, they also have limited access to culturally safe and appropriate health care, which results in hesitance to attend medical appointments and enter hospitals for treatment.

The AIHW report on endometriosis shows a lower rate of endometriosis-related hospitalisations among First Nations people: 2.5 per cent compared with 5.9 per cent of all female hospitalisations. This means they are not receiving the treatment they need for endometriosis.

The National Aboriginal Community Controlled Health Organisation (naccho.org.au) is the peak body for Aboriginal and Torres Strait Islander health. There are over 300 clinics across Australia. They deliver holistic, comprehensive and culturally competent primary healthcare services in a culturally sensitive way to improve health outcomes for Aboriginal and Torres Strait Islander peoples.

Jean Hailes Foundation for Women's Health (jeanhailes.org.au) also has culturally appropriate resources for First Nations people and supports health practitioners in providing health care respectfully.

A First Nation's endo warrior advocating for health: Sara's story

Sara is a proud Aboriginal and Torres Strait Islander woman, employment advocate and business entrepreneur. She is a strong Kamilaroi woman from the Moree Plains of Northern New South Wales.

I have been privileged to mentor Sara for many years. She has been a director of Printing with Purpose (a printing firm owned by Aboriginal women+) since 2019 and spent two years as the director of Aboriginal Economic Development in the Victorian Government Department of Jobs, Skills, Industry and Regions.

Sara has been working in the recruitment and employment industry for 20 years, and her mission is to provide 'culturally appropriate employment, recruitment, and training services for Aboriginal and Torres Strait Islander people'.

Sara never loses sight of her Aboriginal culture and where she came from. Her early family life has made her determined to facilitate change; challenge the drivers of hardship and poverty; and improve outcomes for individuals, their families, Aboriginal and Torres Strait Islander communities, and society as a whole through the dignity and economic stability of work.

Sara is an endo warrior who, now aged 40, is advocating for her own daughters who are suffering symptoms. Sara started experiencing symptoms of pelvic pain, cramping and heavy menstrual bleeding when she started menstruating at age 12. She had her first endometriosis surgery following an ectopic pregnancy.

So many doctors made me think I was making up the pain and bleeding. I underwent 20+ clean-out and explorative surgeries before eventually having a hysterectomy at 32. I am glad I had had all my children by 30.

Unfortunately, Sara's mum wasn't well during her childhood and, being the third child of four and the first girl, she 'didn't have a conversation about periods with me; she was going through so much trauma in her own life,' she said.

So, I, on that first day of my period, thought that I was bleeding to death and ran home from school unsure as to what was going on. I had no other support around. We didn't have family; I didn't have sisters. We didn't have support services. As a 12-year-old girl going to the toilet and, all of a sudden, you've got blood everywhere, you know, your first fear is that you're dying.

I spoke to Mum, and she just said, 'Now you know that the next 20, 30 years of your life is going to be hell on earth'.

Now I am 40, a mother of four, and advocating so strongly for my own daughters on their journey. They're aged 22 and 16, and the health system in Melbourne is completely the opposite of what my mum and I had growing up.

Sara notes, with frustration, that little has changed in the treatment options.

I've got a 16-year-old girl who haemorrhages for 10 days every month, and their answer is to put her on the pill. That's not an answer. She's an elite sportsperson trying to do year 10. I still feel we are at that exact point where I was, getting diagnosed and there's no solution, there's no answers, there's no reason.

Through my own experiences, I know where to take my girls. I'm not prepared to be pushed aside like I was. So, I think there are things in place as you get older, but I don't think there are things in place for those kids getting diagnosed early on. It's still a very grey area.

There is a genetic link — my mum and all of my aunties had been living with this disease for their whole lives. The first GP that we went to told me basically to get all my family out of the way before I was 25 because they couldn't guarantee what would happen. But, based on my mother's experience in medical history, it didn't look good...

Sara was a ward of the state after moving from home to South Australia:

I was just shy of 16. I was living under the state's care and had fallen pregnant, and they sent me to the medical centre numerous times because I was haemorrhaging. They just kept telling me that I was miscarrying, basically because I was a young Aboriginal kid who, in their eyes, shouldn't have been pregnant at all. They just kept sending me home, sending me home, sending me home, telling me that you could bleed for anywhere up to three months, and that's normal. Come back if anything changes from that. The pain got worse.

Nobody really again took me seriously until, eventually, I was rushed to emergency, pretty much vomiting, really unwell, high fevers. One doctor finally did a scan and realised that I wasn't miscarrying and that I had an ectopic pregnancy, which had ruptured my fallopian tube.

When she returned to school, she was 'determined to stay out of trouble, get through until you're 18 years old, leave the public care system... There was no genuine care. There were no supports. Nobody sat down with me, came to doctor's appointments, and told me anything I should be doing.'

I was left to go to appointments by myself. I was left to try and advocate for myself that this pain was not normal. Doctors told me, 'It's normal to bleed this much. Some people get lucky and have three days, and others are just like you. You're not abnormal. This is normal. You just need to learn to live with it.'

I moved to Melbourne at 16. Life had become pretty unbearable living in Adelaide, and I decided, working with the Department of Human Services back then, that I would come to Melbourne and finish year 12 here, and that there were more opportunities work-wise to come out of Victoria. So I got permission to leave South Australia and enter Victoria, met my [future] husband, who was fantastic, and we had our first child. And while he didn't get it, he genuinely knew something wasn't right. I was very blessed to be able to fall pregnant with all of my children. The problem was that my uterus didn't want to stay pregnant. It would start contracting from about 23 weeks, they'd need to induce the baby. So I've never actually been able to carry a baby to term, and I've never been able to go naturally into labour.

After her first baby, Sara was told the endometriosis should be better; instead, it came back with a vengeance.

It's like it had been in hibernation, like a bear that hadn't eaten all winter. The first period that I got after having my firstborn was probably one of the worst I'd ever had in my life; I was losing clots the size of ... probably the bottom of a bottle. Again, people would say to me, that's just normal. That's your body just realigning.

I could fall pregnant, the rest of my insides were riddled with endometriosis and scar tissue, so it was almost like trying to get the foreign object out. I had heard you were meant to have this, I guess, bliss of nine months of not having endometriosis symptoms because you don't have a period. I got maybe three months of that. I still bled. So I still had a period with spotting, regular spotting throughout my pregnancy, which was the same for my mum.

I've now got scars all over my stomach just from different keyhole surgeries. When I had appendicitis, they wouldn't do keyhole surgery again because the surgeon was too scared of what he was going to hit. So I ended up with the old school really big appendicitis scar.

The more debilitating part of it is not the bleeding, it's actually the pain that goes with it. I was bedridden, and now I'm watching it with my own girls like I watched my own mum. Endometriosis pain consumes your whole world. It consumes your everything.

You start to plan your life around eight days of menstruating, from ten days of bleeding to four days in bed. You know, how do you live a life where, for four days a month you are bedridden? How do you explain that to people? How do you explain that to employers? How do you explain that to boyfriends? I know, being 17, 18 years old, how do you explain to somebody who has no idea what's going on in your world that you are stuck in bed and you can't see why I'm in pain, you can't physically, I don't have a broken leg, I don't have a broken arm. I'm just absolutely bent over. I would be feeling like I'm giving birth. It is just the most debilitating pain, and I would not wish it on my worst enemy.

Sara's call to action is 'Education in schools, in workplaces, in the health system'.

Too many Aboriginal and Torres Strait Islander people are waiting well over 12 months to have a laparoscopy to get a diagnosis, to treat their pain. Think about how this impacts our mental health system and our schooling system, and you want to understand why the gap isn't closing. Well, situations like this where I've got a 16-year-old kid who can't go to school because she's in too much pain and she's haemorrhaging and there's no solution. But, yet, you wonder why our education gap is not closing, or our employment is not closing, or our health management isn't closing. Even for a kid from a relatively well-to-do Aboriginal family, with private health insurance, they are long on delays and short on answers.

It is so much worse for people from First Nations communities across our country. I'm not talking about the kids who are in the system and the kids who don't have access to any real help...I am talking about proud Aboriginal and Torres Strait Islander girls and women who can't get the care they need. It breaks my heart.

A search for answers: Lisa's story

Lisa is the founder and CEO of Astrid, Australia's first female-led dispensary, clinic and plant wellness destination. She's a multi-award winner, including CommBank Young Hero of the Year and Top 10 Trail Blazing Pharmacist of the Year, and has been featured in *Forbes*, *Women's Agenda* and *SmartCompany*.

I have the best job in the world. I help patients improve their life and wellbeing by using natural and alternative medicines. Seeing patients' lives transform using medicinal cannabis as a treatment is so rewarding and so incredible. As a female-led business, 60 per cent of my patients are women. I've had the privilege of seeing first-hand how medicinal cannabis has helped women suffering from endometriosis, pelvic pain, chronic pain, insomnia and anxiety.

My parents are Vietnamese immigrants who arrived in the late 1980s by boat in search of a better life. As a first-generation daughter, I've always been taught respect. It is embedded in our DNA as Vietnamese children. I am the second eldest of almost 25 cousins who all live in the south eastern suburbs of Melbourne, Victoria.

My whole life, my parents worked hard. They came here with nothing but the clothes on their back—so hard work, resilience and tenacity are embedded into our complex, multi-faceted Australian-Vietnamese upbringing.

At the age of nine years old, in grade 4, I was at school when I got my period for the first time. But I didn't know what a 'period' was. I panicked and tried to hide it. It was such a young age to be menstruating, and I was so scared because I thought I had done something wrong.

I didn't want to tell my teachers, but, of course, I couldn't hide the blood and my parents found out. I told them I thought it was eczema, so don't worry. But my mum told me no, it's not eczema and she told me what a period was. She taught me how to use pads and how the bleeding would come every month. I remember feeling her sadness as she told me. I knew she was sad that I had to learn how to be a 'woman' when I was still only a child. I cried that night after my mum put on my pad.

I'm married to the most wonderful, loving husband ever and last year we embarked on our fertility journey. I was diagnosed with PCOS, but the cause of my infertility is unknown. I know it sounds horrible, but I always knew that I would eventually have fertility issues—I just knew.

We went to multiple fertility doctors, changing fertility specialists not once, not twice, but three times in a span of

12 months. Each time, we were told different things. Each time, we were expected to do another round of IVF. Each IVF round was more injections, more hormones, more pessaries, more blood tests, more tablets. It was exhausting, and there were so many times when I didn't know if I could keep doing another round.

My body started to change. The hormones made me gain weight. The doctors thought I was immunocompromised because I have eczema and said I had 'increased natural killer cells', so they made me take prednisolone [a corticosteroid that treats inflammation] for weeks on end—to the point where my face turned into the shape of the moon—moon face being one of the major side effects of steroid medication.

My skin became itchy and dry from the constant up-and-down changes in hormones. I also started losing hair, and I cried in the shower every time I saw more hair go down the drain.

I had miscarriage after miscarriage. And each time, the doctors couldn't give me answers. One of the last phone calls with the nurses—from a clinic that I won't name—lasted for three minutes. She called to let me know the transfer didn't result in a viable pregnancy, and sounded so impersonal, and I could feel her disingenuity through the phone—it was like she was reading from a script to fake empathy. I felt numb on the inside.

As a Vietnamese person, I can say we aren't very good at tact. I remember a very core moment that almost broke me—and I believe will stay with me for the rest of my life. I was eating my cousin's birthday cake, and my uncle came up to me and said, 'You shouldn't eat that; you're so fat now'.

I remember freezing and feeling waves of anger, sadness and defeat overtake me. I brushed it off because, of course, in Vietnamese culture, we're taught to respect our elders and not talk back. But he kept going: 'You should eat less, you've gained so much weight.' At this point, my CEO brain switched into gear and I replied calmly and respectfully: 'I'm just letting you know that I've just experienced multiple miscarriages, I've just had another IVF failed cycle a few weeks ago and I've been on hormonal medication that has caused weight gain', thinking he'd back off after I had given him a logical response.

But he kept going... I heard his daughter, my cousin, to my left say, 'Dad, you're being so mean'. In that moment, I froze. I kept repeating, 'It's from the medications'. As the words slipped out of my lips over and over again, I felt so much anger. Anger that I had to even defend myself. Anger that women are expected to bounce back after they've lost an embryo, let alone multiple embryos. Angry that there is an expectation for women to look a certain way without regard for what stage of life they're going through.

I felt myself break down. In my moment of vulnerability, I turned around to grab my husband and I broke down in uncontrollable sobs in his arms. It was the first time I've ever cried in front of my big Vietnamese family.

Last week, I underwent hysteroscopy and laparoscopy surgery. I have found myself a new fertility doctor who is kind, patient and empathetic. And one of the first things she told me when she saw me for the first time was: 'I can almost guarantee that you've got endometriosis, and this is probably the cause of your infertility.'

The surgery went well and very smoothly—and sure enough, post-surgery, my fertility doctor tells me that I've had two very blocked fallopian tubes, and she's found some signs of endometriosis. She told me that my infertility has been environmental (that is, blocked tubes and endometriosis, alongside PCOS) and said now we could try naturally. I felt so happy and so relieved at that moment I almost cried—not just because we could try naturally, but simply because we finally have answers.

And with infertility, half the pain and frustration is just not knowing or no-one being able to give you answers and feeling like an experiment. In that moment, speaking to my fertility specialist and seeing the genuine light and care in her eyes—I felt human again.

My fertility journey isn't over—we are still praying for a miracle baby, but I can feel in my heart, that we are close. I hope that my story inspires more women to speak up and advocate for themselves—not just for their uterus health but also for their emotional and mental health.

Dr Maryam Moradi on increasing awareness of endometriosis

Maryam is originally from Iran and was granted Australian permanent residency as a 'distinguished talent' in 2021, and our nation is richer for it. She has a Bachelor of Science in Midwifery, a Master of Science in Midwifery Education, and a PhD in Medical Sciences. Maryam also has a Diploma in Sexual and Reproductive Health Research.

Maryam's PhD was focused on the experiences of women+ with endometriosis: 'We developed an endometriosis impact questionnaire to measure the long-term impact of endometriosis [2010–2014] on different aspects of women+'s lives.' The 'Impact of endometriosis on women+'s lives: a qualitative study' was groundbreaking and is a highly cited study (Moradi et al., 2014).

'Endometriosis was really under-researched. I was lucky to work with Professors Melissa Parker, Anne Sneddon, Lopez Violeta and David Ellwood. It was a great experience', she recalls. So much so that the band got back together to research and develop 'The Endometriosis Impact Questionnaire' designed to measure the long-term impact of endometriosis.

> *This questionnaire has been translated into over 10 languages and is used internationally. It highlights the varied impacts of endometriosis on different aspects of life, such as marital relationships, social life, physical and psychological wellbeing, and financial stability.*

Dr Moradi is concerned by the ongoing barriers women+ face in getting a timely diagnosis and effective treatment, particularly in conservative or non-English speaking communities. She says it is 'Critical we are committed to increasing awareness, education and support for patients and health professionals in the broader community, but particularly in non-English-speaking and culturally diverse communities'.

Dr Moradi highlights the challenges young women+ face when they are prescribed contraceptive pills for endometriosis in culturally or religiously conservative environments.

Intersectionality and inclusion in care **249**

> *Increasing awareness among parents and communities is so important, and explaining this is a medicine. We need to provide comprehensive information to support understanding in different languages; this is crucial in navigating these challenges.*
>
> *It is also important to emphasise a multidisciplinary health care approach. For example, recent studies emphasise the importance of lifestyle interventions, such as diet, regular physical activity, avoiding cigarette use, alcohol and [getting] good sleep. For example, an anti-inflammatory diet that increases the intake of fruit, vegetables, omega-3 fatty acid organic food and decreases consumption of meat, ultra-processed and fatty food helps manage endometriosis symptoms.*

She says the evidence supports that 'complementary therapies, herbal therapies, acupuncture and massage therapies assist in controlling endometriosis symptoms. The patient benefits from multidisciplinary care.'

She notes her recent work on the federal government–funded Endometriosis Management Plan (Endo-MP) for GPs, led by Professor Danielle Mazza AM and Monash University: 'We heard from patients, general practitioners and other medical stakeholders, and endometriosis organisation representatives and several schools. The needs of girls and women+ from CALD [culturally and linguistically diverse] backgrounds are included.'

LGBTQIA+

LGBTQIA+ is an initialism for lesbian, gay, bisexual, transgender, intersex, queer/questioning, and asexual. Individuals may also choose to describe their experiences of their gender, sexuality and physiological sex characteristics as non-binary, not identifying exclusively as male or female, and pansexual, for whom gender is not a factor in attraction.

Endometriosis does not discriminate. Unfortunately, the health and research sectors do.

There is little enough education about menstruation, let alone endometriosis in schools. In a heterosexual world, where it is assumed you are straight and cis-gender, finding information about endometriosis is even more challenging if you are lesbian, transgender or gender diverse.

Endometriosis can present unique challenges for gender-diverse couples. For those living with endometriosis, there are limited treatments and considerations for painful sex within same-sex couples. There is stigma in accessing gynaecological care and unease with the penetrative pelvic examination through transvaginal and transrectal ultrasounds.

For diagnosis, reliance on 'sub-fertility' as an indicator of endometriosis is clearly not relevant. As for treatment, gender-diverse and lesbian women+ often don't feel comfortable being prescribed a contraceptive pill when they are seeking pain relief. Other treatments like IUDs can be perceived as invasive and may not be favoured.

There can be a lack of understanding and support from healthcare providers. Many providers are not well-versed in the needs of gender-diverse patients with endometriosis. This can lead to dismissive attitudes, inappropriate language and inadequate care. Worse, discrimination against non-heterosexual people can be confronting.

Transgender and non-binary individuals may face barriers in obtaining treatments like hormone therapy or hysterectomy that could help manage endometriosis symptoms. The combination of endometriosis-related pain and gender dysphoria can take a significant toll on mental health.

Endometriosis can impact sexual function and fertility, which may be especially difficult for gender-diverse couples to cope with. Limited resources and services exist, mainly because endometriosis itself is so poorly understood. LGBTQIA+ couples are not included in many resources for people experiencing painful sex.

Research studies do not actively recruit gender-diverse participants. As a result, there are data gaps regarding the prevalence of endometriosis and other conditions among LGBTQIA+ individuals.

Be aware

The Pelvic Pain Foundation of Australia has an education session for trans and gender-diverse teens and their families. Online PPEP Talk sessions (see page 206) are evidence-based programs run in a supportive, empowering and inclusive environment. They are suitable for teens aged 18 and under and are inclusive of all genders, sexualities and identities.

Be prepared

See Chapter 5 for more on physical and internal examination and ultrasound so you know what to expect. Consent should always be sought by the medical practitioner or physiotherapist—and given by you—for physical and internal examination and ultrasound. Know you can stop at any time.

Seek out LGBTQIA+-friendly clinicians and look at LGBTQIA+ Health Australia and Thorne Harbour Health, in the resources section.

Living with endo as part of the LGBTQIA+ community: Max's story

Max Jahufer is a proud father, husband, transgender man and endo brother. He is also an actor; writer; and owner of FutureStudio Agency, a creative digital and marketing agency, and Roaring Tribe, a film and TV production company dedicated to developing content that elevates diversity and amplifies authenticity.

Max's journey has not been without its challenges. He struggled his whole life with extreme pelvic pain and periods prior to transitioning. In his early 30s, he was diagnosed with stage 4 endometriosis, which has significantly impacted his daily life for as long as he can remember.

252 The Australian Guide to Living Well with Endometriosis

Despite the physical and emotional toll, Max's determination never wavered. His struggle with his gender identity further complicated his relationship with endo, a daily reminder of a body he didn't want to inhabit.

In 2020, he decided to transition to become and align with the gender he has always felt he has been. The hormone treatment helped with his dysphoria and his symptoms, improving his ability to cope with the disease that he shares his body with. This experience has deepened his empathy and fuels his desire to advocate for better health care and awareness for those within the LGBTQIA+ community living with endometriosis.

I got my first period around the age of 12, accompanied by nausea, tiredness, heavy, heavy, heavy bleeding, just all of those generic things they tell you are normal, but now I know they are not. I think because both my mum and my grandmother had exactly the same basic history, it was normalised in our family.

I think the advice that they were given was very much the same as today ... it was just to have a baby. It all goes away when you have a baby.

Endometriosis and periods were never spoken about at school.

We spoke about it very much at home. For me, I think, at school, it was almost an embarrassment. Without a doubt, education about abnormal menstruation and endometriosis needs to be provided in schools. It has such personal and severe implications for everyday life. They've got to be discussing this stuff with kids very early on, boys and girls, regardless, because it's a problem that impacts over half of our society. I noticed at school that my friends didn't struggle like I did. I then sort of realised, okay, so I'm the one who's actually different. It's not normal to have those symptoms.

Telling people about the painful symptoms and heavy bleeding became an issue later on in life:

... doing a job that required me to be in the office all the time; the majority of my bosses, probably 95 per cent of my bosses, were male. I never had issues talking about it, but when you're approaching your boss in their office and going, 'Hey mate, I need to take a day off because of XYZ', all of a sudden, it gets all awkward. It shouldn't be—they have a wife, after all. There was just no understanding. Telling someone at work you are struggling physically shouldn't make anyone awkward. Discussing menstruation health and endometriosis needs to be normalised.

Max is used to awkward conversations around his sexuality and is grateful to his family for their support.

I was actually really blessed. My mother and grandmother are very open-minded and modern in their ways and who they are. So I was always very much encouraged just to be who I was, you know, regardless of anything, but also just those conversations were quite normal in a household, even with my dad and my grandfather. It wasn't taboo at all, which is weird from a European background, especially a Portuguese one.

It's been an interesting journey, I think. When trans people discuss their journeys, it's all very unique to the person, so I don't think you'll ever hear two trans stories that are the same ... I think it's more about not who I felt I was externally, which didn't match my feelings internally and that was the struggle ... I did go through the majority of my life, from my early teens through to my late 20s identifying as a gay female because there was no-one else to identify with or see myself in around me. Being trans wasn't spoken about. There was no-one really in a high-profile position that you could sort of look up to or even in the media to sort of go, 'Maybe that's what I am'.

It took me a little while to decide I'm not even a lesbian, I actually identify as male. So once I sort of worked through that, it was really good. I think it's funny because my endometriosis symptoms disappeared just after I moved to Sydney when I was 32. They disappeared out of nothing. No-one could figure out why. I think that was a time in my life when I started to acknowledge my internal feelings about who I really was.

I decided to transition in 2020 during COVID. I don't know why; I just did it. So I entered COVID as a female and left COVID as a male, which is quite interesting. But, look, it's been an amazing, interesting, fulfilling, scary journey. But I think it's now helped me decide that I didn't choose to become Max. I always have been, so it was just finding Max.

His endo symptoms have settled, but despite this, Max still gets some pelvic pain:

I have flare-ups every now and then, which aren't great. But I know how to manage them and stuff like that, which is really good. Nevertheless, I guess, yeah, the testosterone did help with that management. Obviously, it will never go away, but it's helped with that. And, who knows, maybe me sort of living my more authentic self again could really help with stress management.

Max recently married Paris, who has 'mild endo and polycystic ovaries, the double whammy. Unfortunately, she had a few issues during our IVF treatment with the polycystic because they are prone to hyperstimulation.'

Two years after the transition, Max became a father to Windsor. 'I'm Daddy. It was amazing and terrifying at the same time. He's just a little parrot. He'll just walk around and say and do exactly what you do. It is so very cute. It is unconditional love, as well. There's no judgement.'

PART VI
Take action
Global efforts

CHAPTER 18

What's the future of endo research and policy?

Once endometriosis becomes part of your life, it impacts every aspect of it. You have heard some inspiring lived experiences full of resilience and hope for the future.

How can you help yourself and others? Advocate, influence, educate and empower. One of the most impactful things you can do is take part in medical, social and scientific research.

National Endometriosis Clinical Scientific Trials Registry

The National Endometriosis Clinical and Scientific Trials (NECST) Network, an Australian Government initiative, is one project that came out of the 2018 NAPE. This is a research network made up of a group of clinicians, healthcare providers, scientists, patients and consumer representatives who are determined to fill the gaps in endometriosis research to improve patient outcomes and our understanding of this condition.

A major research project being undertaken by members of the NECST Network is to generate Australia's first long-term health dataset on those living with endometriosis, its symptoms and related conditions (including adenomyosis). This project is called the NECST Registry and Biorepository and will enable data and biosamples (e.g. tissue, bloods, urine) to be collected from endometriosis patients throughout their journey from diagnosis to medical treatment, surgery and beyond. The long-term data collected during this project will, over time, help record a detailed picture of the disease—its effects, symptoms, treatments, care and outcomes.

If you would like to participate or find out more about the NECST Registry, please visit unsw.edu.au/research/necstnetwork/registry.

Professor Jason Abbott on the need for multi-disciplinary support for people with endometriosis

Professor Jason Abbott is the co-convenor, along with Professor Gita Mishra, of the WCE to be held in Sydney, May 2025. I am honoured to serve on the organising committee. He is a professor of obstetrics and gynaecology at the University of New South Wales and works in an interdisciplinary team with colorectal surgeons, urologists, anaesthetics, as well as plastic and cardio-thoracic surgeons for extensive extra-pelvic endometriosis and believes in holistic care.

He is Chair of the National Endometriosis Clinical and Scientific Trials (NECST) Network, Australia, directs the Gynaecological Research and Clinical Evaluation (GRACE) research group and is a member of the Endometriosis Advisory group to the Australian Government.

Professor Abbott's advice to those suffering persistent pelvic pain, who have a working diagnosis of endometriosis or a person caring for someone going through the diagnosis or treatment process is to 'educate yourself and know your options'. If you're not happy with the medical advice you're given or you feel dismissed, not heard or not provided options you're comfortable with, he advises you to get a second or third opinion.

Once you have a name for your pain or a proposed treatment presented to you, don't rush. You have time to make decisions... It may be that you are trying hormone treatments first, and sometimes you need to try more than one or trial a medication for a few months to give your body time to adjust. That may resolve your most impactful symptoms without surgery. Sometimes pelvic physiotherapy and other allied and complementary treatments are of benefit.

It is important to be patient with pain. Remember, your pain has been winding up like a clock for five, ten, 15, even 20 years. It isn't going to resolve itself immediately. It needs time to unwind and break habits, including muscle tension, and you need to allow your body time to recondition and readjust.

Endometriosis and adenomyosis impact your body 'upstream and downstream'. As well as your pelvic floor, you can have IBS, even IBD [inflammatory bowel disease], [in which case] dietary change may help. You have the psychological burden of carrying the heavy weight of chronic pain, which is ever present and defines your sense of self.

He suggests psychological and mental health support is important for recovery, along with physical interventions. In his extensive experience, Professor Abbott has seen many women+ worsen as a result of treatments 'and not just surgery or invasive interventions, but from medication and physiotherapy triggering symptoms, even counselling can be detrimental if the practitioner lacks the right expertise'.

He implores those living with endometriosis to consider it an 'evolving disease', and understand that the impacts change over decades. It may be painful sex was your most impactful symptom, then it becomes fertility challenges and heavy menstrual bleeding. Then you're managing menopause symptoms through pharmacology treatments to suppress estrogen, naturally due to age, or a result of hysterectomy.'

He urges women+ to be part of the research, to give of themselves to help learn answers for their own treatment and future generations:

Longitudinal studies, where data is gathered over time, is so crucial. It shows us how the endometriosis lesions and other symptoms change, even in individuals. It shows what works for whom and helps us learn why.

Professor Abbott urges women+ who have improved, whose symptoms are managed, and who are less burdened by endometriosis to continue with research studies. 'These patients are the greatest key to learning why some people get better and some get worse.'

Parliamentary Friends of Endometriosis Awareness

Australia and the endometriosis community around the world owe a great deal to some 'angry birds'. I can call female politicians that because I served as a Member of Parliament myself from 1996 to 2002.

On 28 March 2017, motivated by the suffering of her friend Barbara Long and now ACT Labor MP Caitlin Tough, the then Labor Member of Parliament for Canberra, Gai Brodtmann, became the first MP to call for the end to the silence about endometriosis and raise its impact on women+ in the federal parliament. She noted this to be one of the most taboo issues of women+'s health—endometriosis had been ignored, just like its sufferers, for too long.

In a 90-second statement that went viral on Facebook, Gai spoke up about 'misdiagnosis myths, operations, hysterectomies in their 20s, endless operations, lost opportunities, impact on mental health, the cost, the pain, and the daily struggle to take control of their lives'.

She brought the endometriosis groups together to advocate for and inform the development of NAPE. This was the catalyst for change. On 5 December 2017, the Parliamentary Friends of Endometriosis Awareness was founded by Gai and then Liberal MP Nicolle Flint, who was living with endometriosis, and Liberal MP Nola Marino, whose daughter Kylie was finally diagnosed in her 30s.

At the launch, Gai said: 'We are well overdue for acknowledgement of this insidious disease; the physical cost, psychological cost, the professional cost, to these women+ and their families and loved ones.'

Then Minister for Health and Aged Care, the Hon. Greg Hunt, apologised to generations of endometriosis sufferers on behalf of all previous governments, and said: 'On behalf of all of those in parliament and all of those who have been responsible for our medical system, I apologise. This condition should have been acknowledged at an earlier time in a more powerful way and will never be forgotten again.'

I asked the Hon. Greg Hunt to reflect on the Coalition's commitment to endometriosis and his apology. He shared that he 'realised there was no agenda and focus on this area, so we set out to give it funding and a plan. I thought the apology was a necessary and critical step to awareness and recognition.'

Then Prime Minister Scott Morrison and his wife Jenny shared their experiences and the impact of endometriosis on their fertility journey. Nola Marino has raised her own daughter Kylie's challenges with endometriosis in parliament on many occasions, and she is current co-chair of the Parliamentary Friends of Endometriosis Awareness with the Labor Member for Bendigo, Lisa Chesters, both of whom are proactive and vocal advocates for endo warriors.

National Action Plan on Endometriosis

Since 2018, the Australian Government has committed $87.2 million to the NAPE's three pillars: clinical management and care; research; and awareness and education. It has directed the funding to improve access to medical imaging, for clinicians to reduce diagnosis delays, to primary care support, research and the endometriosis community. However, while these commitments are welcome and very long overdue, endometriosis and pelvic pain remain underfunded and under-resourced.

NAPE has funded some initiatives, including EndoZone (see page 279), research like LongSTEPPP (see page 205), Medical Imaging and Imagendo (see pages 54 and 55), education, and the GP Management Plan.

Endometriosis and pelvic pain clinics

I was delighted to be with the Hon. Ged Kearney MP for the announcement of the first 20 endometriosis and pelvic pain clinics on 21 March 2023 (which increased to 22 six months later). It received non-partisan support from Shadow Minister for Health, Senator the Hon. Anne Ruston, Libby Coker, Larissa Waters, Susan Templeman, Zali Steggall, Lisa Chesters, Sophie Scamps, Monique Ryan, Sally Sitou and Alicia Payne, representing the Liberal Party, the Nationals, the Greens and independent MPs.

The clinics receive $200000 per year for four years for endometriosis care and patient management to improve diagnosis time frames and direct patients to appropriate pain management. The funds can also be used for advanced training qualifications, further study, additional practice staff (e.g. allied health, nurse navigators), enhanced referral pathways with local providers or equipment purchases.

The aim is to improve patients' access to diagnostic, treatment and referral services for endometriosis and pelvic pain, and support them with resources, care pathways and networks. There is a very broad approach to patient services, with some clinics providing multidisciplinary care, with physiotherapists and dietitians, and others coordinating integrated care with psychologists and other independent health providers in allied and complementary health services.

The 'Endo 22' clinicians meet monthly to discuss innovation and resources, and listen to guest speakers and a broad range of health and wellbeing practitioners.

Last, and unfortunately least, the community organisations that support the endometriosis community, not as patients but as sufferers of endometriosis, received $2 million through the Increasing Awareness of Endometriosis Amongst Priority Populations for a mentor program to support those newly diagnosed with endometriosis and to help employees and employers navigate workplace discussions through guidelines. This funding was announced in January 2024, six months after the five-year NAPE expired.

I was honoured to attend the announcement of funding for priority populations with the Hon. Ged Kearney MP and Associate Professor Anusch Yazdani in January 2024 at the Endometriosis and Pelvic Pain Clinic at Benowa Medical Centre on the Gold Coast. QENDO (an organisation that advocates for people with endometriosis and other pelvic health-related conditions) President Anita Fung and Australian Coalition for Endometriosis Chair Jessica Taylor spoke, along with me and a couple of friends I invited, Kayla Itsines and Kylie Brown, who spoke about their lived experiences.

Creating change at the policy level: Nicolle's story

In 2017, Nicolle Flint, then the federal Liberal member for Boothby in the Federal Parliament, heard her Labor colleague Gai Brodtmann in the House of Representatives raise issues about endometriosis. They both recall Nicolle chasing Gai out of the chamber, introducing herself as 'brand new' and wanting to work with her to do something with their respective Minister and Shadow Minister for Health about the disease.

They became co-founders of Parliamentary Friends of Endometriosis Awareness in the Australian Parliament. They worked together to advocate for the development of NAPE and proudly welcomed new funding for research, awareness and treatment in specialised clinics.

Nicolle retired from the federal parliament before the 2022 election, mainly due to her endometriosis symptoms. She has announced that she is going to re-contest the seat of Boothby for the Liberal Party because her endometriosis is now more under control.

I think, like most women with endometriosis, I was probably always having symptoms. I thought that my period pain was normal. We know that is very, very common. I didn't even seek help for that because there was no education or awareness. I thought that taking a packet of Panadeine every time I got my period was normal.

In large part, thanks to the work of former Labor member for Canberra Gai Brodtmann in raising endometriosis in the Parliament, this led to my own diagnosis of endometriosis.

Together, we founded the Parliamentary Friends of Endometriosis Awareness. I give full credit to Hon. Greg Hunt, the Minister for Health, for supporting us.

With the self-diagnostic tools that are now available, we will continue to see women getting or self-diagnosing at least a lot sooner in a way that I wasn't able to because the information did not exist until 2018, when the NAPE was launched.

Nicolle recalls it was 'about 10 years before I got my actual diagnosis because it was always about my bowel. I still have extensive endo lesions there. I've had two major surgeries, but I have been concerned about doing more, knowing that many women+ have very serious complications, ending up with a colostomy bag; that's always been my biggest fear, really.'

Other symptoms are bloating linked to her menstrual cycle, and Nicolle was also diagnosed with coeliac disease.

All of the endo warriors out there should know that getting gluten out of your diet and trying to bring down inflammation in that way is one of the key things that is recommended. And so when I did that, it was quite life changing. And I had a big reduction in my symptoms for probably five or six years.

During that time, I was elected to the federal parliament in a marginal seat. You work so hard, and you often neglect yourself and your health because you are so busy trying to do your job to the best of your ability with a huge amount of scrutiny and all of the stuff that goes with being in politics.

My symptoms progressively got worse, and again, it was always about my bowel pain and being bloated because, again, I thought that my period pain, which from time to time was excruciatingly severe and debilitating, was so bad that I thought I would pass out. It got to the point where I was feeling so terrible that I thought, okay. Clearly, there's something wrong with my bowel; this is what women traditionally have gone through. It's not endo, it's not my periods, it's something else.

I encourage everyone to use the RATE tool developed by RANZCOG [see page 32], as a self-diagnosis tool. I'm proud that this was among the resources I helped create when I was in federal parliament. I also want to acknowledge the foundational work of the Jean Hailes Foundation for Women's Health with NECST and EndoZone, which is part of The University of Adelaide and has great resources and information.

You have to be your own advocate. There is a great need for more education for GP specialists, health practitioners, physios and nurses. We've come a really long way, but there's so much more to do. To be your best advocate, educate yourself as much as possible.

We do know it's an inflammatory disease. We do know it is often in the pelvic region and it can result in complex gynaecological issues.

For me, my pain did not change after laparoscopic surgery, and this is the case for many women. It is important to manage people's expectations, but also reassure people that it's okay. You can keep looking for different treatments if your surgery doesn't relieve your pain. Everyone is different.

Medications affect women differently. The Pelvic Pain Foundation of Australia has a fantastic resource on its site, which goes through all the different pain relief medications. It goes through all of the different medications that are used to treat endo generally. I share many really simple fact sheets with so many women who are still on their journey and trying to get proper help.

Now that the five-year National Action Plan on Endometriosis has expired, we need to focus on a new NAPE. We need to keep working on the health system, expand the endometriosis and pelvic pain clinics, and learn more and support access to holistic, person-centred treatments, like complementary medicines, pelvic physiotherapy, acupuncture, yoga and Pilates. Self-care treatments like this really make an impact.

Global endo efforts

Australia's universal health care system (Medicare) is far from perfect, but we are fortunate to have a stable health and hospital system. It is challenged and stretched, with bed shortages resulting from nurse shortages, funding shortages and so on becoming endemic after a pandemic.

Even in a nation with subsided access to health care, where 55 per cent of the population have private health insurance, women+ have and continue to face diagnostic delays and lack of informed care for endometriosis, persistent and chronic pelvic pain, and other general health conditions and diseases.

We have established the fact that even frontline healthcare providers often fail to recognise that debilitating pelvic pain is not a normal condition. These diagnostic delays hinder timely access to available treatment options, hormonal therapies and devices as well as surgery.

Internationally, there are notable medical knowledge gaps in developing, low- and middle-income countries, particularly those without robust women+'s rights. The World Health Organization (WHO) is working with 'multiple stakeholders, including academic institutions, non-state actors and other organisations that are actively involved in research to identify effective models of endometriosis prevention, diagnosis, treatment, and care'.

While primary health practitioners (the ones at the entry level to health systems) should be trained in and aware of endometriosis symptoms, diagnostic screening, physical examinations and basic management, they lack the effective tools for symptom identification, let alone ongoing management.

While significant strides are being made globally to address endometriosis through awareness campaigns, research funding and integrated care models, challenges remain. Multidisciplinary teams need to be equipped with the necessary skills and resources for early diagnosis and effective treatment of endometriosis.

Continued and strong individual and community advocacy for increased research and treatment funding and improved healthcare access is essential for enhancing outcomes for those affected by this debilitating condition. We are fortunate to have the first NAPE and must not be complacent about the second, third, fifth, tenth and twentieth iterations of future NAPEs.

Australia is a world leader in the endometriosis health, wellbeing and research sectors. We owe it to the pioneers of NAPE, including Gai Brodtmann, Nicolle Flint, Greg Hunt, Anne Ruston and Ged Kearney, to continuously improve support for the one in seven Australian women+ who will be diagnosed with endometriosis by their 50th birthday.

Women+ with endometriosis need to work with those at the forefront of the world's efforts to improve outcomes through treatment research until a cure is discovered and dispensed to the estimated 190 million girls and women+ who deserve to live the life they want without pain.

Here are some of the global efforts to foster living well with endometriosis.

World Endometriosis Society (WES)

WES (endometriosis.ca) is the global organisation for endometriosis and adenomyosis clinical practice, research, education and advocacy. WES is the go-to organisation for all involved in caring for women+ with endometriosis and adenomyosis. It facilitates research in the aetiology, pathogenesis and pathophysiology of endometriosis and adenomyosis to discover a cure and prevent endometriosis. WES advocates for recognising endometriosis and adenomyosis as a health priority with a major burden on the woman+, her family, workplace and society. WES coordinates broad collaboration with all stakeholders in endometriosis and adenomyosis. It has a membership of diversity (professions, region, gender, etc.), embraces all nations and continues to grow.

World Congress on Endometriosis 2025 Sydney

Hosted by WES (www.wce2025.com.au/org-committee), the biannual congress aims to advance the understanding of patient treatment, patient care and the causes and consequences of the disease on the lives of countless women+.

I am proud to serve on the organising committee and as chair of the Patient Liaison Committee with the rockstars of the endo health and research sector. I particularly wish to acknowledge the co-convenors, Professor Jason Abbott and Professor Gita Mishra, along with the Immediate Past President of the WES Professor Luk Rombauts. Please take a look at the other endometriosis sector representatives representing Australia on the world stage and looking after the endometriosis community in Australia.

World Endometriosis Organisations (WEO)

Founded in 2017, WEO (endometriosis.org/support/world-endometriosis-organisations-weo/) is a peak organisation for endometriosis community groups and works to encourage greater emphasis on collaboration, improve relationships with all stakeholders, share expertise to advance skills and knowledge, contribute to the research, and identify new and innovative opportunities to enhance connectivity and positive contributions to the cause. I want to acknowledge New Zealander Deborah Bush, WES Board Trustee and Principal founding member of the World Endometriosis Organisations for her tireless work.

The gift of philanthropy

Philanthropy Australia defines philanthropic donations as 'the giving of money, time, information, goods and services, influence and voice to improve the wellbeing of humanity and the community'. These donations are made through private or public ancillary funds, sub-funds and giving circles, testamentary or other legacy trusts and dedicated financial vehicles from individuals and families.

Donations are crucial in advancing medical research, enabling breakthroughs that can significantly improve health outcomes. Here are some notable examples of philanthropic gifts in the field of medical research for endometriosis.

Wilson Foundation

As a private family foundation based in Australia, the Wilson Foundation is dedicated to leveraging its philanthropic efforts to enhance outcomes for women+ with endometriosis. Its focus includes advancing early diagnosis, strengthening the evidence for integrated treatment options to alleviate pain, and expanding new models of care that improve health outcomes. It is currently funding two trials in Australia.

In the area of new models of care, the Wilson Foundation are partnering with the Julia Argyrou Endometriosis Centre (JAECE) at Epworth to fund an endometriosis nurse coordinator. This role enables JAECE to expand its multidisciplinary team to support more patients. Additionally, the Wilson Foundation is funding a project officer at JAECE to develop and disseminate resources based on the centre's multidisciplinary care model.

EndoChill trial at The University of Adelaide

This novel trial will evaluate the efficacy and safety of cold water therapy as a treatment for the pain associated with endometriosis. It will involve breathwork, cold water immersion and meditation.

In addition, the trial will examine how cold water immersion affects psychological status, endometrial lesion characteristics, the autonomic nervous system, endocrine system responses and innate immune responses.

EndoCann trial at Western Sydney University

This novel trial will evaluate the efficacy and safety of medicinal cannabis as a treatment for the pain associated with endometriosis. It will investigate the endocannabinoid system, its role in inflammation and endometriosis, and its response/non-response to medicinal cannabis. As well as the cost/benefits of medicinal cannabis as a treatment for endometriosis, the use of transvaginal ultrasound for determining lesion staging and progression, and cognitive functioning after the use of medicinal cannabis for endometriosis.

Eden Foundation

Established by Simon and Anna Ainsworth in 2008, the Eden Foundation is a philanthropic trust and charitable branch of Sydney's Eden Gardens. With daughter Lily living with endometriosis, since 2022, they have committed around $616000 to research to find answers for the one in seven women+ diagnosed by their 50th birthday.

The Lambert Initiative

In 2015, Count Financial founders Barry and Joy Lambert donated $33 million to Sydney University to research cannabis treatments, which established the Lambert Initiative for Cannabinoid Therapeutics.

The Lambert Initiative is currently developing novel cannabinoid-based treatments for a range of different diseases and conditions. It is also involved in education, community outreach, science-based advocacy and policy issues relating to medicinal cannabis. Currently, the Lambert Initiative supports the research of more than 30 clinicians, academics, postdoctoral fellows, research assistants and students and has many national and international research collaborators.

Acknowledgements

Endometriosis is invidious and insidious. Its impact is unjust and unfair.

I first heard the word *endometriosis* from the late, great Professor David Healy in 1997.

He was a prominent figure in the field of obstetrics and gynaecology, particularly known for his significant contributions to the understanding and treatment of endometriosis. He had recently become the head of reproductive medicine at Monash University and was a founder of Jean Hailes for Women's Health in 1992.

I had been elected to the Parliament of Victoria the year before. My electorate covered Monash University, Monash Hospital, Monash IVF, Monash Institute of Medical Research and Prince Henry's Institute of Medical Research—the latter two merged in 2014 to form the Hudson Institute of Medical Research.

At the time, I was chair of the government's health policy committee and went on to be Parliamentary Secretary for Health and Human Services. From a women+'s health and gender equity perspective, the sheer numbers of those living with endometriosis and the devastating impact on them staggered me. Of course, the baby I was carrying is also among the one in seven Australian women+ diagnosed with endometriosis by their 50th birthday.

Professor Healy passed away in 2012, leaving a legacy marked by his unwavering commitment to improving women+'s health through research and education. His influence continues to resonate within the medical community, particularly among those dedicated to advancing the understanding of endometriosis.

In recognition of his contributions, WES established the David Healy Award to honour individuals who have made significant advancements in endometriosis research and treatment. It was an honour to see his friend and mentee, Professor Luk Rombauts, then president of WES, present an award in David's name at the WCE in Edinburgh in 2023 and in Sydney in 2025.

Jean Hailes for Women's Health is a national not-for-profit organisation dedicated to improving women+'s health across Australia through every life stage. I acknowledge the untiring dedication of the namesake's daughter, Janet Michelmore AO, now patron, who serves on the Australian Government Endometriosis Advisory Group.

Charity founders include the eminent Professor Peter Rogers (University of Melbourne), Professor Susan Davis AO (Monash University), Dr Elizabeth Farrell AM (current medical director of Jean Hailes for Women's Health), the late Professor Henry Burger AO, whom I first met when he was director of Prince Henry's Institute from 1990 to 1998 and then emeritus director of Hudson Institute, and the aforementioned late Professor David Healy. I attended the opening of the clinic in 1992, which was officiated by Hazel Hawke. The team does amazing work and has supported both my daughters.

I also acknowledge the dedication of CEO Dr Sarah White, who serves on the National Women's Health Advisory Council and the Therapeutic Goods Administration's Women's Health Products Group.

I met Professor Euan Wallace, now the secretary of the Victorian Department of Health, when he arrived at Monash from Edinburgh in 1996. He is a wonderful person. He was the Carl Wood Professor of Obstetrics and Gynaecology at Monash University and was formerly Safer Care Victoria's inaugural CEO. He has driven the endometriosis and gender pain gap agenda with the Inquiry into Women's Pain and the Victorian Pelvic Pain Symposium.

I also want to pay tribute to my own gynaecologist and obstetrician, Dr Tony Lawrence, who has looked after me for over 30 years, delivered my three children and, indeed, 'made' the last one at Monash IVF. He was a founding doctor at the first endometriosis clinic in Melbourne in 1991, with IVF pioneer Professor Carl Wood, Dr Bruce Downing, Dr Mac Talbot, Dr Mary Wingfield and Dr Nick Lolatgis.

The Endometriosis Association of Victoria drove the establishment of the original clinic and much of the early awareness of the condition. The co-founders of the organisation, Ros Wood (who remains active with endometriosis.org) and Lorraine Henderson, wrote a book with journalist Robyn Riley (she's the current medical director for News Corp's *Herald Sun*) called *Explaining Endometriosis* (1994). Professor David Healy gave me a copy of the book. I know Ellie Angel-Mobbs's mum, Barbara, still has her copy.

In 1999, this clinic became part of Epworth Health. The legacy continues with the recent establishment of the Julia Argyrou Endometriosis Centre at Epworth (JAECE). I am privileged to call Julia my friend. She and her husband, Michael Argyrou, are tireless in their advocacy and financial support to actively assist those living with endometriosis and invest in research.

Dr Sofie Piessens, a gynaecologist, also earns a mention for her work in bringing specialised ultrasound techniques to Australia to diagnose deep infiltrating endometriosis with transvaginal ultrasound. She was 'encouraged' to go to Brazil to study this in 2009 by her husband, Professor Luk Rombauts; Associate Professor Jim Tsaltas, a gentleman and scholar who has cared for Brianna and me and is based at Epworth and Melbourne IVF; Associate Professor Martin Healey, from Royal Women's, Mercy and Epworth; and the late Professor Peter Maher, who passed away in May 2023.

I have been honoured to serve on the organising committee for the WCE, held in Sydney in May 2025, and to be appointed chair of the Patient Liaison Committee, in collaboration with Jessica Taylor, chair of the Australian Coalition for Endometriosis and CEO of QENDO.

I pay homage to co-convenors of WCE 2025 Professor Jason Abbott and Professor Gita Mishra, and their fellow eminent colleagues on the WCE committee:

- Dr Rebecca Deans, Professor Caroline Ford, Dr Erin Nesbitt-Hawes, Dr Cecilia Ng (University of New South Wales)
- Professor Grant Montgomery, Associate Professor Anush Yazdani, Dr Brett McKinnon, Dr Sally Mortlock (University of Queensland)
- Professor Roger Hart (University of Western Australia)
- Professor Louise Hull (University of Adelaide)
- Associate Professor Mike Armour (Western Sydney University)
- Associate Professor Subhadra Evans, Dr Antonina Mikocka-Walus (Deakin University)
- Professor Caroline Gargett, Professor Luk Rombauts (Monash University)
- Associate Professor Peter Rogers (University of Melbourne)
- Dr Leesa Van Niekerk (University of Tasmania).

In closing, my sincerest thanks to the endo warriors who shared their intimate lived experiences to empower others and ease their journeys.

To the rockstars, eminent clinicians and researchers who generously shared their expertise, I am incredibly grateful, and I thank you on behalf of the endo community.

I thank the Wiley team, Lucy Raymond, who is the driving force behind this book becoming a reality, and the editing team, Leigh McLennon, Chris Shorten, Ingrid Bond, and Melanie Dankel, with marketing magic provided by Renee Aurish.

I am privileged to have shared the journey with endo and adeno through my beautiful, brave, resilient daughter Brianna. I want to acknowledge the support of my family—my ever-patient husband, Marcus, always there beside me on life's adventures. John Lennon said, 'Life is what happens to you while you're busy making other plans'. This book wasn't in our life plan, and I am grateful to my three children who have supported and encouraged me as I typed. I owe some quality 'Nanree' time to my three beloved grandchildren.

My amazing parents, Pat and Terri, have been my greatest inspiration and devoted champions. They raised me and my five siblings to be fiercely loyal to each other, help those who need a hand up, be empathetic, respect all people, see the individual and pursue injustices.

While writing this book, I cared for my friend, neighbour and business partner, Paul, as he fought leukaemia. He lost his battle just after his 55th birthday, and I dedicate this book to his memory and will fulfil my promise to be a strong role model for his daughter.

You can find further information and interviews with book contributors and gender equality mediation services at my websites www.advisorygovcorp.com.au/ and http://endoencompass.com.

Resources

I recommend EndoZone, Jean Hailes for Women's Health and Julia Argyrou Endometriosis Centre as the pre-eminent sources of empirical, evidence-based information for those living with endo symptoms, a diagnosis of endometriosis or associated inflammatory and gynaecological conditions.

EndoZone

EndoZone (endozone.com.au) is a digital platform about all things endo and has been developed by researchers, health experts and health informatics specialists in conjunction with Australia's endometriosis associations. It has specific resources for clinicians, parents, teachers, employers and employees. The website has information on symptoms, diagnosis, treatment and surgery, as well as work-life balance and self-management.

It was established with funding from the Australian Government and Jean Hailes for Women's Health. It is based at the Endometriosis Research Group at Robinson Research Institute, The University of Adelaide.

Jean Hailes for Women's Health

Jean Hailes for Women's Health (jeanhailes.org.au) has been at the forefront of empirical, evidence-based information and medical treatment for endometriosis and menopause since 1992. Visit the website for general information about symptoms, causes, management, fertility and more.

Julia Argyrou Endometriosis Centre at Epworth

JAECE (epworth.org.au/our-services/endometriosis-centre) provides clinical and patient information resources, webinars and support focused on a holistic approach to patient care that covers all aspects of treatment: social, emotional and physical wellbeing. Established in 2022 with philanthropic gifts from the Argyrou family and other donors, it focuses on research and person-centred integrated care.

World Endometriosis Organisations

World Endometriosis Organisations (endometriosis.org) is a network of organisations who have pooled their collective power together to improve outcomes for women+ with endometriosis. The WCE (www.wce2025.com.au) is a global event focused on endometriosis.

General information

There are a number of organisations that can provide general information on endometriosis and how it affects a range of domains.
- Australian Patients Association: www.patients.org.au
- Consumer Health Forum: chf.org.au
- Australian Government Health Direct: www.healthdirect.gov.au/search-results/endometriosis
- Australian Women and Girls' Health Research Centre: public-health.uq.edu.au/research/awaghr-centre
- Better Health Channel: www.betterhealth.vic.gov.au/health/conditionsandtreatments/endometriosis
- Endometriosis, World Health Organization: www.who.int/news-room/fact-sheets/detail/endometriosis
- Endometriosis.org has a handy glossary: endometriosis.org/glossary.

Heavy menstrual bleeding and periods

- Share the Dignity www.sharethedignity.org.au
- The Women's Royal Hospital Victoria: www.thewomens.org.au health-information/periods/endometriosis
- Bleed Better: www.bleedbetter.org
- EndoZone: www.endozone.com.au/heavy-bleeding-during-your-period
- Jean Hailes: www.jeanhailes.org.au/uploads/09_HP-tools/Heavy_menstrual_bleeding_tool.pdf

Tracking symptoms

There are numerous tools you can use to track your symptoms, which is highly recommended so your health professional can see patterns and have evidence of prolonged symptoms. Free tools you can use to do this include:

- The Raising Awareness Tool for Endometriosis (RATE) developed by RANZCOG with a multidisciplinary group: www.cognitoforms.com/f/zYpsFXGgJU6rZe8W0IVotA?id=131
- QENDO app: www.qendo.org.au/qendo-app
- Heavy Menstrual Bleeding Bayer: www.mybodymyway.com.au/know-your-flow
- Period ImPact and Pain Assessment (PIPPA): www.canberrahealth services.act.gov.au/pippascreening

Endometriosis support groups

Despite the struggles we've outlined that many women+ have experienced in seeking an accurate diagnosis, there is support available for women+ with pelvic pain, heavy bleeding and all the symptoms that tell you your pain is not normal. Some of those resources include the following:

- ACE peak body for endometriosis: acendo.com.au
- Endo Active: endoactive.org.au
- Endometriosis Australia: endometriosisaustralia.org
- Endometriosis WA: www.endometriosiswa.org.au

- Pelvic Pain Foundation Australia: pelvicpain.org.au
- QENDO (patient resources and free management app): qendo .org.au

Endometriosis online peer support groups

- Tasmania Endometriosis Support Group: facebook.com/groups/ 433797400120644
- Australian and New Zealand Women With Endometriosis Support Group: facebook.com/groups/425058554296380
- Endometriosis Victoria support group: facebook.com/groups/ 190048611055868
- Melbourne Endometriosis Sisters: facebook.com/groups/ MelbEndoWarriors
- Endometriosis Western Australia: facebook.com/EndometriosisWA
- QENDO: facebook.com/qendo/groups

More on the website www.endoencompass.org

Resources for adenomyosis

Adenomyosis (when tissue grows into the wall of the uterus) is an added burden for many women+ with endo. There is support for this specific condition.
- Adenomyosis Australia: adenomyosis.org.au
- Health Direct information on adenomyosis: www.healthdirect .gov.au/adenomyosis
- Jean Hailes for Women's Health information on adenomyosis: www.jeanhailes.org.au/health-a-z/ovaries-uterus/adenomyosi

Advocacy

Change can sometimes be slow but it doesn't happen without the dedication of people who care about the issue. One place advocacy can start is with your local member.
- Members of the Australian Parliament and Senators: www.aph .gov.au/Senators_and_Members/Contacting_Senators_and_ Members

- Australian Government Directory (www.directory.gov.au/) has information about departments, agencies, as well as state and territory government directories:
  - Australian Capital Territory: www.directory.act.gov.au
  - New South Wales: www.service.nsw.gov.au/nswgovdirectory
  - Northern Territory: nt.gov.au
  - Queensland: www.qld.gov.au/about/contact-government/contacts/government-directory
  - South Australia: www.sa.gov.au/directories/government
  - Tasmania: directory.tas.gov.au/cgi/access.pl
  - Victoria: www.vic.gov.au/victorian-government-directory
  - Western Australia: www.wa.gov.au/information-about/wa-government

Endometriosis and pelvic pain clinics

The Australian Government has funded specialist GP endometriosis and pelvic pain clinics to improve patients' access to diagnostic, treatment and referral services, build the primary care workforce to manage endometriosis, and improve access to new information and care pathways to help build a patient-centred, multidisciplinary team that empowers self-care between medical appointments. See page 263 or visit: www.health.gov.au/ourwork/endometriosis-and-pelvic-pain-clinics#current-endometriosis-and-pelvic-pain-clinics

Education for young girls and women+

The more we can learn about menstrual health and what is considered 'normal', the more empowered women+ will be to advocate for their health. Here are some resources that get the right conversations started.
- PPEP Talk for Schools (providing education in schools, sports programs and for trans and gender-diverse teens; see also page 206): www.pelvicpain.org.au/ppep-talk-schools-program
- LongSTEPPP research (join the long-term research study on endometriosis: see also page 205): redcap.mcri.edu.au/surveys/?s=WJWMJT73JRT9YEM8
- What about ME? Menstrual Health and Endometriosis (New Zealand): www.periodhealth.nz

Education and guidelines for health, allied and integrative practitioners

- Pelvic Pain Foundation of Australia: www.pelvicpain.org.au/about/for-health-professionals
- Australian Commission on Safety and Quality in Healthcare Heavy Menstrual Bleeding Clinical Standard: www.safetyand quality.gov.au/standards/clinical-care-standards/heavy-menstrual-bleeding-clinical-care-standard
- Australasian Society for Ultrasound in Medicine Education: www.asum.com.au/education
- Endometriosis Ultrasound Worksheet: www.asum.com.au/files/public/Others/Endometriosis-ultrasound-worksheet.pdf
- EndoZone Clinicians Centre: www.endozone.com.au/clinicians
- Endometriosis education for primary health providers developed by RANZCOG: acquire.ranzcog.edu.au/mod/page/view.php?id=13314
- RANZCOG Australian Endometriosis Guideline: ranzcog.edu.au/news/australian-endometriosis-guideline
- Jean Hailes for Women's Health: www.jeanhailes.org.au/health-professionals
- FODMAP diet: www.monashfodmap.com/online-training/dietitian-course
- Information for clinics: www.monashfodmap.com/shop
- European Society of Human Reproduction and Embryology ESHRE guideline endometriosis: eshre.eu/Guidelines-and-Legal/Guidelines/Endometriosis-guideline
- Fertility Society of Australia and New Zealand: www.fertilitysociety.com.au/health-professionals
- Vagenius (accredited by RACGP, RANZCOG, EndoZone): www.vageniustraining.com
- Matilda physiotherapy resources to optimise surgical outcomes: www.matilda.health/clinicians
- RACGP Women's Health general guidelines (not endo specific): www.racgp.org.au/clinical-resources/clinical-guidelines/key-racgp-guidelines/view-all-racgp-guidelines/preventive-activities-in-general-practice/reproductive-and-womens-health; www.racgp.org.au/clinical-resources/clinical-guidelines/guidelines-by-topic/view-all-guidelines-by-topic/women-s-health

- Mental Health First Aid: www.mhfa.com.au/our-courses
- Pain Australia: www.painaustralia.org.au/painaustralia-health-professionals/painaustralia-education-training

Infertility

As we've seen throughout the book (and in many of the personal stories women+ have shared) that endometriosis can create fertility issues in women+ and, for some women+, the only hope to end their pain is often a hysterectomy. Understanding your fertility and the supports out there can empower you to take control of your journey to become a parent (or not).

- Fertility Society of Australia and New Zealand www.fertility society.com.au/patient-centred-care
- Health Direct information about fertility: www.healthdirect.gov .au/about-infertility
- My Doctor on female infertility: mydr.com.au/babies-pregnancy/ female-infertility

Family planning clinics

These clinics offer support for all reproductive and sexual healthcare needs, pregnancy counselling, reproductive and sexual health information and support. Medicare rebates and bulk-billing may apply to consultations at family planning clinics.

- ACT: Sexual Health & Family Planning ACT (SHFPACT): www .shfpact.org.au
- NSW: Family Planning Australia: www.fpnsw.org.au
- Northern Territory: Family Planning Welfare Association of NT Inc.: www.fpwnt.com.au
- Queensland: True Relationships and Reproductive Health: www .true.org.au
- South Australia: SHINE SA: shinesa.org.au
- Tasmania: Family Planning Tasmania: fpt.org.au
- Victoria: Sexual Health Victoria: shvic.org.au
- Western Australia: Sexual Health Quarters: shq.org.au

Fertility Society of Australia and New Zealand

The Fertility Society of Australia and New Zealand (fertilitysociety .com.au) represents health professionals working in reproductive medicine in Australia and New Zealand. The website has a wealth of resources on IVF, donors, surrogacy, infertility and more.

Grief in pregnancy, fertility, birth and perinatal death

Miscarriage, stillbirth and perinatal death are heartbreaking and isolating experiences for women+ and couples. An unsuccessful IVF round is also the loss of a much-wanted baby.

- The Pink Elephant support network provides information and guidance on your journey, founded Sam Payne, an endo warrior: www.pinkelephants.org.au
- Pregnancy, Birth and Baby: www.pregnancybirthbaby.org.au/ miscarriage
- PANDA Planning, starting, raising a family www.panda.org.au

Financial stress resources

Endometriosis unfairly penalises women+, which affects their finances. Medical appointments, treatments, surgeries, medications and missed work due to illness can have a detrimental effect on women+'s financial lives. Improving your financial literacy can set you on a path to better manage.

- Beyondblue: www.beyondblue.org.au/mental-health/financial-wellbeing
- Good Shepherd: goodshep.org.au/services/fih
- Zahra Foundation: zahrafoundation.org.au/financial-counselling
- 1800 RESPECT: 1800respect.org.au/services/services-overview/ money
- Women's Information and Referral Exchange Inc' Victorian based with online information: www.wire.org.au/category/topics/ financial-wellness

Food and FODMAP

Chapter 12 covered the benefits of eating foods that work with your body and symptoms. A Low-FODMAP diet could help with symptoms such as bloating and gas.

- Monash University: www.monashfodmap.com/about-fodmap-and-ibs
- Starting the FODMAP diet: www.monashfodmap.com/ibs-central/i-have-ibs/starting-the-low-fodmap-diet
- Dietitians Australia: dietitiansaustralia.org.au/diet-and-nutrition-health-advice
- Naturopaths and Herbalists Association of Australia: nhaa.org.au
- How Not to Die: NutritionFacts.org

Medicinal cannabis

Rachel Payne, member of the Legalise Cannabis Victoria party, outlined some the benefits and barriers to use medicinal cannabis to control pain in Chapter 6. Find out more:

- Medicinal cannabis: www.odc.gov.au/medicinal-cannabis
- TGA Cannabis Hub: www.tga.gov.au/products/unapproved-therapeutic-goods/medicinal-cannabis-hub

Natural therapies

Herbs, acupuncture and osteopathy are just a few examples of natural therapies that can help manage endo pain.

- Naturopaths and Herbalists Association of Australia (NHAA): nhaa.org.au
- Herbal medicine, Department of Health and Human Services: www.betterhealth.vic.gov.au/health/conditionsandtreatments/herbal-medicine
- Australasian Association of Ayurveda: www.ayurved.org.au/
- Australian Acupuncture and Chinese Medicine Association (AACMA): www.acupuncture.org.au/about-aacma
- Endometriosis and natural therapies, Jean Hailes: www.jeanhailes.org.au/health-a-z/endometriosis/endometriosis-natural-therapies

LGBTQIA+

If you are part of the LGBTQIA+ community, you may feel that there are not a lot of supports out there for your unique circumstance. The following links can offer information and connections.

- LGBTQIA+ Health Australia (resources on everything from mental health and suicide prevention to disability inclusion): lgbtiqhealth.org.au
- LGBTQIA+ and Endo, Endometriosis WA: www.endometriosiswa .org.au/im-seeking-support/endometriosis-and-gender-diversity
- FemXX Health: www.femxx.health/post/lgbtqia
- LGBTQIA+ resources, Nancy's Nook: nancysnookendo.com/ lgbtqia-resources
- Rainbow Health Australia (focused on training, advocacy and education across a range of LGBTQIA+ issues): rainbowhealth australia.org.au
- Thorne Harbour Health (a rich resource covering multiple topics on LGBTQIA+ health as well as community-led programs): thorneharbour.org

Mental health and wellbeing national support numbers

Living with chronic pain can have implications for your mental health and wellbeing. Help is always out there and having mental health support should be a cornerstone of your treatment.

- Body Image Movement and Embrace Kids: bodyimagemovement .com
- Butterfly National Helpline (for support with eating disorders or body image concerns): 1800 33 4673 or visit www.butterfly .org.au
- MindSpot (online tool offering confidential and personalised mental health support): mindspot.org.au/assessment
- Lifeline (crisis support and suicide prevention services available via phone, text message or online chat): 13 11 14

- 13Yarn (counselling and crisis support for Aboriginal and Torres Strait Islander peoples): 13 92 76
- Kids Helpline (counselling for kids, teens and young adults aged between five and 25 available via phone and online chat): 1800 551 800
- Suicide Call Back Service (phone and online counselling for people affected by suicidal thoughts or suicide available via phone, online chat and video calls): 1300 659 467
- MensLine Australia (counselling service offering support to men available via phone, online chat and video calls): 1300 789 978
- SANE Helpline (counselling, peer support, online groups and community forums for people aged 18+ with complex mental health needs and their family, friends and carers): 1800 18 7263
- Beyond Blue (brief, confidential counselling services available via phone or online chat): 1300 22 4636
- Qlife (anonymous LGBTQIA+ peer support and referral available via phone and online chat) 1800 184 527
- Open Arms (counselling for anyone who has served at least one day in the Australian Defence Force and their families) 1800 011 046
- Thorne Harbour Health LGBTQIA+ counselling: thorneharbour .org/services/lgbtiq-mental-health/counselling

Medical costs and rebates

Australia has a universal health system, and you can find out what's covered by Medicare and how to enrol if you're an eligible Australian or New Zealand citizen, Australian permanent resident, applying for permanent residency or have a temporary resident covered by a ministerial order: servicesaustralia.gov.au/medicare.

- Australian Government Medical Costs Finder (find costs for general and specialist services in Australia): health.gov.au/ resources/apps-and-tools/medical-costs-finder
- Healthdirect (find GPs, specialists and other healthcare providers near you): healthdirect.gov.au/australian-health-services
- Privatehealth.gov.au (learn more about private health insurance and compare policies): privatehealth.gov.au/footer/ costsfinder.htm

More on the website www.endoencompass.org

Medical misogyny

'End gender bias survey results–summary report', Australian Government: www.health.gov.au/womens-health-advisory-council/resources/publications/endgenderbias-survey-results-summary-report?language=en.

Ovarian cancer

Ovarian cancer is a general term used to describe a cancerous (malignant) tumour starting in one or both ovaries.

- Signs to look out for: www.ovariancancer.net.au/about-ovarian-cancer/symptoms
- Symptom diary (a tool to easily record symptoms): www.datocms-assets.com/102334/1691392879-symptom-diary.pdf
- How doctors test and diagnose ovarian cancer: www.ovariancancer.net.au/about-ovarian-cancer/diagnosis-and-results

Pain and pelvic pain

Endometriosis comes with numerous potential symptoms, one of the biggest being pain. These organisations support the management of pain and can direct you to a specialist for specific care.

- Pelvic Pain Foundation of Australia, a founding member of the Australian Coalition for endometriosis: www.pelvicpain.org.au
- Endometriosis: www.pelvicpain.org.au/endometriosis-post
- For teens: www.pelvicpain.org.au/find-support/for-teens
- For women+: www.pelvicpain.org.au/for-women
- Find a professional: www.pelvicpain.org.au/find-support/find-a-health-professional/
- Pain Australia: www.painaustralia.org.au/pain-services-directory/pain-directory
- Meg Odgers Pelvic Pain and Sexual Pain Resources: endohelp.com.au/wp-content/uploads/2023/08/Pelvic-Pain-and-Sexual-Pain-Resources-website.pdf

Physiotherapy, wellbeing and exercise

Chapter 11 talks about the benefits of exercise on overall health and some of the types of exercise that can be better suited to people with endometriosis. If you're looking for more physical health options to explore, try the following:

- Kayla Itsines Exercise for Endo (explore gentle movement for pain relief): sweat.com/blogs/wellbeing/endometriosis-awareness-month-workout
- Pelvic Physiotherapy Vagenius (resources on pelvic stretching and breathing): vageniustraining.com
- Pelvic stretches: www.vageniustraining.com/resources/pelvic-stretches
- Breathing to calm your farm (pelvic, bowel and brain): www.vageniustraining.com/resources/relaxed-breathing
- Post-surgery avoiding lifting and straining: www.vageniustraining.com/resources/avoiding-lifting-and-straining
- Continence Foundation of Australia (information on bladder and bowel control): www.continence.org.au/who-it-affects/women/female-pelvic-floor-muscles
- Physiotherapy Matilda app (focuses on four core pillars, including movement, for self-care before and after surgery for conditions like endometriosis): www.matilda.health
- Transcendental Meditation: tm.org.au/
- Wim Hof method (breathing and cold therapy): www.wimhofmethod.com
- Mindfulness: www.healthdirect.gov.au/mindfulness

Relationships

Conversations around sex with your partner when sex is painful can be difficult. There are supports out there that can arm you with information, plus aids that can help find the right balance between pleasure for all parties and comfort.

- 1800Respect (you have a right to respect and safety in all your relationships): 1800respect.org.au/healthy-relationships
- Society of Australian Sexologists: societyaustraliansexologists.org.au

- Relationships Australia: www.relationshipsvictoria.org.au/counselling
- Australian Psychological Society: psychology.org.au

Sex and intimacy

Try some of the following:
- Painful sex guide (learn why sex might be painful for you): pelvicpain.org.au/painful-sex-women
- The sync set (conversation starters on topics related to sex, dating and intimacy): itsnormal.com
- OHNUT (a set of rings that can help you control the depth of penetration; see also page 147): www.pelvicpain.org.au/product/ohnut

Surgery

Australasian Gynaecological Endoscopy and Surgery (AGES) Society has built on its vision to promote the safest and highest standards of clinical and minimally invasive surgical care for women+ through its three tenants of education, surgical training and clinical research: ages.com.au/patient/patient-resources.

The Royal Women's Hospital in Melbourne maintains up-to-date resources on endometriosis, hysterectomy and other relevant information: www.thewomens.org.au/health-information/periods/endometriosis/laparoscopy-and-endometriosis; thewomens.r.worldssl.net/images/uploads/fact-sheets/Hysterectomy-abdominal-280519.pdf; thewomens.r.worldssl.net/images/uploads/fact-sheets/Hysterectomy-total-laparoscopic-280519.pdf

Therapeutic Goods Administration (TGA)

The TGA is Australia's government authority responsible for evaluating, assessing and monitoring products that are defined as therapeutic goods. It regulates medicines, medical devices and biologicals to help Australians stay healthy and safe.
- Medicinal Cannabis Hub: www.tga.gov.au/products/unapproved-therapeutic-goods/medicinal-cannabis-hub
- Report a problem or side effect: www.tga.gov.au/safety/reporting-problems
- Safety alerts: www.tga.gov.au/news/safety-alerts

Workplace, gendernomics

It's important to know your rights and obligations in the workplace.
- Supporting workers with endometriosis in the workplace, Safe Work Australia: /www.safeworkaustralia.gov.au/doc/supporting-workers-endometriosis-workplace
- Flexible working arrangements for employees with disability: www.fairwork.gov.au/newsroom/news/flexible-working-arrangements-employees-disability
- Unreasonable refusal of a support person, Fair Work Commission: www.fwc.gov.au/unreasonable-refusal-support-person
- Occupational health and safety—your legal duties, WorkSafe Victoria: www.worksafe.vic.gov.au/occupational-health-and-safety-your-legal-duties
- Endo can end women's careers and stall their education, The University of Queensland: public-health.uq.edu.au/article/2022/03/endometriosis-can-end-women%E2%80%99s-careers-and-stall-their-education-%E2%80%99s-everyone%E2%80%99s-business
- A survey of leaders living and working with chronic illness, The University of Melbourne: fbe.unimelb.edu.au/__data/assets/pdf_file/0007/4639318/Disclosing_Illness_at_Work_Ghin_Ainsworth.pdf

Research

While endometriosis research is underfunded and often overlooked, there is still some incredible work being done by some talented people. You can read about some of the projects currently running.
- Adelaide Endometriosis Research Group: www.adelaide.edu.au robinson-research-institute/research/research-groups/endometriosis
- Australian Longitudinal Study on Women's Health (ALSWH): alswh.org.au
- The Australian Institute of Health and Welfare (AIHW) Endometriosis report is updated regularly with data on prevalence, hospitalisations and other important information. It is based on data from the ALSWH: www.aihw.gov.au/reports/chronic-disease/endometriosis-in-australia/contents/endometriosis

- Endometriosis Diagnosis Innovation and Treatment group in Melbourne has a mixture of clinical trials and lab-based research leading to a better understanding of factors that lead to the development and progression of endometriosis: www.endometriosis.org.au/projects
- Endometriosis.org provides information on global efforts into endometriosis: endometriosis.org/topic/resources/
- The Gynaecological Research and Clinical Evaluation (GRACE) Unit at Royal Hospital for Women in Sydney undertakes quality women+'s health and benign gynaecological research that will improve the care and outcomes for girls, women+ to live their best and healthy lives: www.unsw.edu.au/medicine-health/our-schools/clinical-medicine/research-impact/research-groups/clinical-research/gynaecological-research-clinical-evaluation-unit
- Hudson Institute of Medical Research is leading medical research into women+'s reproductive health and is home to some of the world's top scientists in endometrial research, focused on developing a non-invasive early diagnostic test, non-surgical and non-hormonal treatment options and to improve detection of infertility in women+ with the disease: www.hudson.org.au/disease/womens-newborn-health/endometriosis
- National Endometriosis Clinical and Scientific Trials (NECST) Registry aims to improve endometriosis care and has a research affiliation with EndoZone Australasian Interdisciplinary Researchers in Endometriosis (AIRE): www.unsw.edu.au/research/necstnetwork/registry
- University of Queensland Institute for Molecular Science has mapped locations of over 30 additional genetic markers for endometriosis risk; identified genes and pathways targeted by some genetic risk factors for endometriosis; developed new cell-based models to study the functions of these genes; and discovered a subset of cells with altered differentiation in endometriosis patients: imb.uq.edu.au/endo
- World Endometriosis Research Foundation collaborates with WES: endometriosis.ca/research/werf/ endometriosisfoundation.org/research/#clinical-studies

References

Introduction

Adenomyosis Australia n.d., Homepage, Adenomyosis Australia, adenomyosis .org.au/about-us/.

Australian Government Department of Health 2018, 'National Action Plan for Endometriosis', Australian Government Department of Health, www.health .gov.au/sites/default/files/national-action-plan-for-endometriosis.pdf.

Australian Institute of Health and Welfare 2023, 'Endometriosis', AIHW, www.aihw.gov.au/reports/chronic-disease/endometriosis-in-australia/ contents/summary.

Endometriosis.org n.d., 'Adhesions', Endometriosis.org, endometriosis.org/ endometriosis/adhesions/.

Endometriosis News 2018, 'Endometriosis and Adhesions', Endometriosis News, endometriosisnews.com/endometriosis-and-adhesions/.

Fan, P & Li, T 2022, 'Unveil the pain of endometriosis: from the perspective of the nervous system', *Expert Reviews in Molecular Medicine*, vol. 5, no. 24, p e36.

Godin, Wagner, Huang, & Bree 2021, 'The role of peripheral nerve signalling in endometriosis', FASEB Bioadvances, vol. 3, no. 10, pp. 802–13.

Maddern, Grundy, Castro, & Brierley 2020, *Expert Reviews in Molecular Medicine*, vol. 24, no. e36.

O'Hara, R, Rowe, H & Fisher, J 2022, 'Managing endometriosis: a cross-sectional survey of women in Australia', *Journal of Psychosomatic Obstetrics and Gynaecology*, vol. 43, no. 3, pp. 265–272.

Royal Australian and New Zealand College of Obstetricians and Gynaecologists 2021, 'Australian Endometriosis Guideline', RANZCOG, ranzcog.edu.au/news/australian-endometriosis-guideline/.

World Health Organization 2023, 'Endometriosis', WHO, www.who.int/news-room/fact-sheets/detail/endometriosis.

Part I: Tune in

Bouaziz, J, Bar On, A, Seidman, DS & Soriano, D 2017, 'The clinical significance of endocannabinoids in endometriosis pain management', *Cannabis and Cannabinoid Research*, vol. 2, no. 1, pp. 72–80.

Chandrakanth, A, Firdous, S, Vasantharekha, R, Santosh, W & Seetharaman, B 2024, 'Exploring the effects of endocrine-disrupting chemicals and miRNA expression in the pathogenesis of endometriosis by unveiling the pathways: A systematic review', *Reproductive Sciences*, vol. 31, no. 4, pp. 932–941.

Cheah, S, Skvarc, D, Evans, S, Van Niekerk, LV & Mikocka-Walus, A 2024, 'Exploring biopsychosocial health outcomes in endometriosis and endometriosis with co-occurring irritable bowel syndrome–a prospective cohort study', Research Square, www.researchsquare.com/article/rs-4505378/v1.

Crump, J, Suker, A & White, L, n.d., 'Endometriosis', *Australian Journal of General Practice*, vol. 53, no. 1–2.

European Association of Urology n.d., 'Chronic pelvic pain', Uroweb, 2024, uroweb.org/guidelines/chronic-pelvic-pain.

Health Direct 2023, 'Adenomyosis–stages, symptoms and treatment', Health Direct, www.healthdirect.gov.au/adenomyosis.

Health Direct 2023, 'Endometriosis', Health Direct, www.healthdirect.gov.au/endometriosis.

International Association for the Study of Pain 2022, 'International association for the study of pain', IASP, www.iasp-pain.org/.

Jean Hailes for Women's Health 2023, 'Adenomyosis fact sheet', Jean Hailes, www.jeanhailes.org.au/resources/adenomyosis.

John Hopkins Medicine n.d., 'Health', John Hopkins Medicine, www.hopkinsmedicine.org/health/conditions-and-diseases/endometriosis.

Leuenberger, J, Kohl Schwartz, AS, Geraedts, K, Haeberlin, F, Eberhard, M, von Orellie, S, Imesch, P & Leeners, B 2022, 'Living with endometriosis: Comorbid pain disorders, characteristics of pain and relevance for daily life', *European Journal of Pain*, vol. 26, no. 5, pp. 1021–38.

Lingegowda, H, Williams, BJ, Spiess, KG, Sisnett, DJ, Lomax, AE, Koti, M & Tayade, C 2022, 'Role of the endocannabinoid system in the pathophysiology of endometriosis and therapeutic implications', *Journal of Cannabis Research*, vol. 4, no. 1, p. 54.

Maddern, J, Grundy, L, Castro, J & Brierley, SM 2020, 'Pain in endometriosis', *Frontiers in Cellular Neuroscience*, vol. 14, p. 590823.

Markham, R, Luscombe, Manconi, F & Fraser, IS 2019, 'A detailed profile of pain in severe endometriosis', *Journal of Endometriosis and Pelvic Pain Disorders*, vol. 11, no. 9, p. 228402651983894.

Maulitz, L, Stickeler, E, Stickel, S, Habel, U, Tchaikovski, SN & Chechko, N 2022, 'Endometriosis, psychiatric comorbidities and neuroimaging: Estimating the odds of an endometriosis brain', *Frontiers in Neuroendocrinology*, vol. 65, p. 100988.

McDonough, LS & Gautieri, A 2018, 'How to make simple homemade cleaning sprays', Good Housekeeping, www.goodhousekeeping.com/home/cleaning/tips/a24885/make-at-home-cleaners/.

Mortlock S, Corona RI, Kho PF, Pharoah P, Seo JH, Freedman ML, Gayther SA, Siedhoff MT, Rogers PAW, Leuchter R, Walsh CS, Cass I, Karlan BY, Rimel BJ; Ovarian Cancer Association Consortium, International Endometriosis Genetics Consortium; Montgomery GW, Lawrenson K, Kar SP. A multi-level investigation of the genetic relationship between endometriosis and ovarian cancer histotypes. *Cell Rep Med.* 2022 Mar 15;3(3):100542. doi: 10.1016/j.xcrm.2022.100542. PMID: 35492879; PMCID: PMC9040176.

Neri, B, Russo, C, Mossa, M, Martire, FG, Selntigia, A, Mancone, R, Calabrese, E, Rizzo, G, Exacoustos, C & Biancone, L 2023, 'High frequency of deep infiltrating endometriosis in patients with inflammatory bowel disease: A nested case-control study', *Digestive Diseases (Basel, Switzerland)*, vol. 41, no. 5, pp. 719–28.

Office on Women's Health n.d., 'Endometriosis', OASH, www.womenshealth.gov/a-z-topics/endometriosis#:~:text=How%20can%20I%20prevent%20endometriosis,uterus%20during%20your%20menstrual%20cycle.

Rowlands, IJ, Abbott, JA, Montgomery, GW, Hockey, R, Rogers, P, & Mishra, GD 2021, 'Prevalence and incidence of endometriosis in Australian women: a data linkage cohort study', *BJOG: An International Journal of Obstetrics and Gynaecology*, vol. 128, no. 4, pp. 657–665.

Women's Health Australia n.d., 'Australian longitudinal study on women's health', Women's Health Australia, alswh.org.au/.

World Endometriosis Society 2021, 'Endometriosis', World Endometriosis Society, endometriosis.ca/endometriosis/.

Xue, Y-H, You, L-T, Ting, H-F, Chen, Y-W, Sheng, Z-Y, Xie, Y-D, Wang, Y-H, Chiou, J-Y & Wei, JC-C 2021, 'Increased risk of rheumatoid arthritis among patients with endometriosis: a nationwide population-based cohort study', *Rheumatology (Oxford, England)*, vol. 60, no.7, pp. 3326–33.

Yang, F, Wu, Y, Hockey, R, International Endometriosis Genetics Consortium, Doust, J, Mishra, GD, Montgomery, GW & Mortlock, S 2023, 'Evidence of shared genetic factors in the etiology of gastrointestinal disorders and endometriosis and clinical implications for disease management', *Cell Reports Medicine*, vol. 4, no. 11, p. 101250.

Yu, Y 2020, 'Understanding endocannabinoid system in endometriosis', Endonews.com, www.endonews.com/understanding-endocannabinoid-system-in-endometriosis.

Part II: Track, tell, test

AusDoc Community Manager 2024, 'A GP guide to persistent pelvic pain', AusDoc, www.ausdoc.com.au/therapy-update/a-gp-guide-to-persistent-pelvic-pain/.

Australian Government n.d., 'Chronic disease GP management plans and team care arrangements, Australian Government, www.servicesaustralia .gov.au/mbs-billing-rules-for-chronic-disease-gp-management-plans-and-team-care-arrangements?context=20.

Australian Government n.d., 'Diagnostic imaging endometriosis MRI medicare benefits schedule - item 63563', Australian Government, www9.health.gov.au/mbs/fullDisplay.cfm?type=item&q=63563.

Better Health Channel n.d., 'Pelvic inflammatory disease (PID)', State Government of Victoria, www.betterhealth.vic.gov.au/health/healthyliving/pelvic-inflammatory-disease-pid.

Better Health Channel 2024, 'Myomectomy', State Government of Victoria, www.betterhealth.vic.gov.au/health/conditionsandtreatments/myomectomy.

Bleed Better n.d., Homepage, Bleed Better, www.bleedbetter.org/.

Bramble, A 2023, 'Everything you need to know about heavy menstrual bleeding (HMB)', WHO, www.who.com.au/lifestyle/health/what-is-heavy-menstrual-bleeding/.

Chalmers, KJ, Catley, MJ, Evans, SF & Moseley, GL 2017, 'Clinical assessment of the impact of pelvic pain on women', *Pain*, vol. 158, no. 3, pp. 498–504.

Crump, J, Suker, A & White, L n.d., 'Endometriosis: A review of recent evidence and guidelines', *Australian Journal of General Practice,* vol. 53, no. 1–2.

Department of Health. Victoria, Australia n.d., 'Iron deficiency anaemia and iron therapy', State Government of Victoria, www.health.vic.gov.au/patient-care/iron-deficiency-anaemia-and-iron-therapy.

Department of Health and Aged Care 2024, 'Historic Medicare changes for women battling endometriosis', Department of Health and Aged Care, www.health.gov.au/ministers/the-hon-mark-butler-mp/media/historic-medicare-changes-for-women-battling-endometriosis#:~:text=In.

Endometriosis Foundation of America 2024, '2024 EndoFound Blossom Award - Bindi Irwin', YouTube, www.youtube.com/watch?v=fnIzWs8GmHU.

Fan, P & Li, T 2022, 'Unveil the pain of endometriosis: from the perspective of the nervous system', *Expert Reviews in Molecular Medicine*, vol. 24, no. e36, p. e36.

Frayne, J, Simonis, M, Lam, A 2024, 'New Australian tool aims to prompt conversations about endometriosis', InSight+, insightplus.mja.com.au/2024/3/new-australian-tool-aims-to-prompt-conversations-about-endometriosis/.

Gater, A, Taylor, F, Seitz, C, Gerlinger, C, Wichmann, K & Haberland, C 2020, 'Development and content validation of two new patient-reported outcome measures for endometriosis: the Endometriosis Symptom Diary (ESD) and Endometriosis Impact Scale (EIS)', *Journal of Patient-Reported Outcomes*, vol. 4, no. 1, p. 13.

Gete, DG, Doust, J, Mortlock, S, Montgomery, G & Mishra, GD 2023, 'Associations between endometriosis and common symptoms: Findings from the Australian Longitudinal Study on Women's Health', *American Journal of Obstetrics and Gynecology*, vol. 229, no. 5, p. 536.e1-536.e20.

Gete, DG, Doust, J, Mortlock, S, Montgomery, G & Mishra, GD 2024, 'Risk of iron deficiency in women with endometriosis: A population-based prospective cohort study', *Women's Health Issues: Official Publication of the Jacobs Institute of Women's Health*, vol. 34, no. 3, pp. 317–324.

Health Direct Australia 2024, 'Chronic fatigue syndrome (Myalgic Encephalomyelitis)', Health Direct, www.healthdirect.gov.au/chronic-fatigue-syndrome-cfs-me.

Hologic 2023, 'Heavy menstrual bleeding market research', Two Blind Mice, www.livecomfortably.au/.

Kiesel, L 2019, 'Endometriosis and anemia', Endometriosis.net, endometriosis.net/clinical/iron-anemia.

ME/CFS Australia, n.d., 'A national perspective for Myalgic Encephalomyelitis', ME/CFS Australia Ltd, mecfs.org.au/.

Mitchell, AM, Rajapakse, D, Peate, M, Chalmers, KJ, Kamper, SJ, Frawley, H, Cheng, C, Healey, M & Lensen, S 2024, 'The "most bothersome symptom" construct: A qualitative study of Australians living with endometriosis', *Acta Obstetricia et Gynecologica Scandinavica*, vol. 103, no. 8, pp. 1625–33.

Moradi, M, Parker, M, Sneddon, A, Lopez, V & Ellwood, D 2019, 'The Endometriosis Impact Questionnaire (EIQ): a tool to measure the long-term impact of endometriosis on different aspects of women's lives', *BMC Women's Health,* vol. 19, no. 1, p. 64.

Munro, CB, Walker, EN, Schembri, R, Moussaoui, D & Grover, SR 2024, 'Periods shouldn't bring any adolescents' world to a full stop. Period. An online survey of adolescents' experience of menstruation', *Journal of Pediatric and Adolescent Gynecology,* vol. 37, no. 1, pp. 18–24.

Neri, B, Russo, C, Mossa, M, Martire, FG, Selntigia, A, Mancone, R, Calabrese, E, Rizzo, G, Exacoustos, C & Biancone, L 2023, 'High frequency of deep infiltrating endometriosis in patients with inflammatory bowel disease: A nested case-control study', *Digestive Diseases (Basel, Switzerland),* vol. 41, no. 5, pp. 719–28.

Nisenblat, V, Bossuyt, PMM, Farquhar, C, Johnson, N & Hull, ML 2016, 'Imaging modalities for the non-invasive diagnosis of endometriosis', *Cochrane Database of Systematic Reviews,* vol. 2, no. 2, p. CD009591.

Piccolo, CL, Cea, L, Sbarra, M, De Nicola, AM, De Cicco Nardone, C, Faiella, E, Grasso, RF & Beomonte Zobel, B 2023, 'Magnetic resonance roadmap in detecting and staging endometriosis: Usual and unusual localizations', *Applied Sciences (Basel, Switzerland),* vol. 13, no. 18, p. 10509.

Piessens, S, Healey, M, Maher, P, Tsaltas, J & Rombauts, L 2014, 'Can anyone screen for deep infiltrating endometriosis with transvaginal ultrasound?', *The Australian & New Zealand Journal of Obstetrics and Gynaecology,* vol. 54, no. 5, pp. 462–8.

Royal Australian and New Zealand College of Obstetricians and Gynaecologists 2022, 'Raising awareness tool for endometriosis (RATE)', RANZCOG, ranzcog.edu.au/resources/raising-awareness-tool-for-endometriosis-rate/.

Stein, M & Sherer D 2024, 'Bindi Irwin what would I tell my younger self', Parade, parade.com/news/what-bindi-irwin-would-tell-younger-self-start-endometriosis-journey-exclusive.

Vagenius Training n.d., 'Resources', Vagenius, www.vageniustraining.com/resources.

Whiting, F 2014, 'Queensland Opposition Leader Annastacia Palaszczuk reveals her private heartache at not having children', The Courier Mail, www.couriermail.com.au/news/queensland/queensland-opposition-leader-annastacia-palaszczuk-reveals-her-private-heartache-at-not-having-children/news-story/6f9e928de3ebd28c136efa3fc72e9538.

Women's Health Australia 2023, 'Women wait for endometriosis diagnosis with multiple symptoms', Women's Health Australia, alswh.org.au/women-wait-for-endometriosis-diagnosis-with-multiple-symptoms/.

Part III: Treat

Anastasi, E, Scaramuzzino, S, Viscardi, MF, Viggiani, V, Piccioni, MG, Cacciamani, L, Merlino, L, Angeloni, A, Muzii, L & Porpora, MG 2023, 'Efficacy of N-acetylcysteine on endometriosis-related pain, size reduction of ovarian endometriomas, and fertility outcomes', *International Journal of Environmental Research and Public Health*, vol. 20, no. 6.

AusDoc Community Manager 2024, 'A GP guide to persistent pelvic pain', AusDoc, www.ausdoc.com.au/therapy-update/a-gp-guide-to-persistent-pelvic-pain/.

Australian Commission on Safety and Quality Health Care n.d., 'Australian Charter of Healthcare Rights', Australian Commission on Safety and Quality Health Care, www.safetyandquality.gov.au/our-work/partnering-consumers/australian-charter-healthcare-rights.

Australian Government n.d., 'Pharmaceutical Benefits Scheme Post-market Review Section Report Stocktake of Pharmaceutical Benefits Scheme subsidised medicines available for endometriosis and related conditions, and comparison of current Australian pharmacological treatment guidelines', Australian Government, www.pbs.gov.au/reviews/endometriosis-and-related-conditions-reports/Endometriosis-medicines-stocktake-and-guideline-comparison-report-November-2022.pdf.

Australian Institute of Fitness 2023, 'The science behind effective massage: Anatomy and physiology', AIF, fitness.edu.au/the-fitness-zone/the-science-behind-effective-massage/.

Becker, CM, Johnson, NP, As-Sanie, S, Arjona Ferreira, JC, Abrao, MS, Wilk, K, Imm, SJ, Mathur, V, Perry, JS, Wagman, RB & Giudice, LC 2024, 'Two-year efficacy and safety of relugolix combination therapy in women with endometriosis-associated pain: SPIRIT open-label extension study', *Human Reproduction (Oxford, England)*, vol. 39, no. 3, pp. 526–37.

Berterö, C, Alehagen, S & Grundström, H 2019, 'Striving for a biopsychosocial approach: A secondary analysis of mutual components during healthcare encounters between women with endometriosis and physicians', *Journal of Endometriosis and Pelvic Pain Disorders*, vol. 11, no. 3, pp. 146–151.

Better Health Channel n.d., 'Ayurveda', Better Health Channel, www.betterhealth.vic.gov.au/health/conditionsandtreatments/ayurveda.

Bourne, KM, Hall, J, Stiles, LE, Sheldon, RS, Shibao, CA, Okamoto, LE, Garland, EM, Gamboa, AC, Peltier, A, Diedrich, A, Biaggioni, I, Robertson, D & Raj, SR 2021, 'Symptom presentation and access to medical care in patients with postural orthostatic tachycardia syndrome: Role of sex', *CJC Open*, vol. 3, no. 12 Suppl, pp. S44–S52.

Bradbury, Z 2024, 'How can body image cause distress for people with endometriosis?', Butterfly Foundation, butterfly.org.au/body-image-concerns-endometriosis/.

Brant, SR & Nguyen, GC 2008, 'Is there a gender difference in the prevalence of Crohn's disease or ulcerative colitis?', *Inflammatory Bowel Diseases*, vol. 14, Suppl 2, pp. S2-3.

Butterfly Foundation n.d., Homepage, Butterfly Foundation, butterfly.org.au/.

Cancer Research UK 2021, 'Epithelial ovarian cancer', Cancer Research UK, www.cancerresearchuk.org/about-cancer/ovarian-cancer/types/epithelial-ovarian-cancers/epithelial.

Choe, J & Shanks, AL 2023, *In vitro fertilization*, StatPearls Publishing.

Chowdary, P, Stone, K, Ma, T, Readman, E, McIlwaine, K, Druitt, M, Ellett, L, Cameron, M & Maher, P 2019, 'Multicentre retrospective study to assess diagnostic accuracy of ultrasound for superficial endometriosis — Are we any closer?', *The Australian & New Zealand Journal of Obstetrics & Gynaecology*, vol. 59, no. 2, pp. 279–84.

Cohen, M, Weisman, A & Quintner, J 2022, 'Pain is not a "thing": How that error affects language and logic in pain medicine', *The Journal of Pain: Official Journal of the American Pain Society*, vol. 23, no. 8, pp. 1283–93.

Conroy, I, Mooney, SS, Kavanagh, S, Duff, M, Jakab, I, Robertson, K, Fitzgerald, AL, Mccutchan, A, Madden, S, Maxwell, S, Nair, S, Origanti, N, Quinless, A, Mirowski-Allen, K, Sewell, M & Grover, SR 2021, 'Pelvic pain: What are the symptoms and predictors for surgery, endometriosis and endometriosis severity', *The Australian & New Zealand Journal of Obstetrics & Gynaecology*, vol. 61, no. 5, pp. 765–72.

Contreras, KM, Buzzi, B, Vaughn, J, Caillaud, M, Altarifi, AA, Olszewski, E, Walentiny, DM, Beardsley, PM & Damaj, MI 2024, 'Characterization and validation of a spontaneous acute and protracted oxycodone withdrawal model in male and female mice', *Pharmacology, Biochemistry, and Behavior*, vol. 242, no. 173795, p. 173795.

Culley, L, Law, C, Hudson, N, Mitchell, H, Denny, E & Raine-Fenning, N 2017, 'A qualitative study of the impact of endometriosis on male partners', *Human Reproduction (Oxford, England)*, vol. 32, no. 8, pp. 1667–73.

Dahiya, A, Sebastian, A, Thomas, An, George, R, Thomas, V & Peedicayil A 2021, 'Endometriosis and malignancy: The intriguing relationship', *International Journal of Gynaecology and Obstetrics*, vol. 155, no. 1, pp. 72–8.

Deakin University 2023, 'Could medicinal cannabis be the answer to the pain of endometriosis?', Deakin University, www.deakin.edu.au/

about-deakin/news-and-media-releases/articles/could-medicinal-cannabis-be-the-answer-to-the-pain-of-endometriosis.

Department of Health and Aged Care: Office of Drug Control n.d., 'Medicinal cannabis', Australian Government, www.odc.gov.au/medicinal-cannabis.

Department of Health & Human Services n.d., 'Herbal medicine', www.betterhealth.vic.gov.au/health/conditionsandtreatments/herbal-medicine.

Dumont, H 2024, '[Sex therapy and support for women and couples]', *Revue de l'infirmiere,* vol. 73, no. 299, pp. 34–5. [French].

Eddie, R 2024, '"Waste of money": Pain specialists challenge endometriosis surgeries', *The Age,* www.theage.com.au/politics/victoria/waste-of-money-pain-specialists-challenge-endometriosis-surgeries-20240731-p5jxz0.html.

Endometriosis Foundation of America 2018, 'Endometriosis stages: Understanding the different stages of endometriosis', Endometriosis Foundation of America, www.endofound.org/stages-of-endometriosis.

Endometriosis.net 2020, 'The benefits of massage', Endometriosis.net, endometriosis.net/clinical/massage-pain.

EndoZone n.d., 'Acupuncture', EndoZone, www.endozone.com.au/treatment/acupunture.

EndoZone n.d., 'Advice for partners', EndoZone, www.endozone.com.au/advice-partners.

EndoZone n.d., 'Physical intimacy', EndoZone, www.endozone.com.au/physical-intimacy.

Engel, GL 1977, 'The need for a new medical model: a challenge for biomedicine', *Science (New York, N.Y.),* vol. 196, no. 4286, pp. 129–36.

Ferrero, S & Barra, F, editors 2020, *Endometriosis: From diagnosis to treatment,* Nova Medicine & Health.

Fertility Society of Australia & New Zealand 2020, 'Code of practice', Fertility Society of Australia and New Zealand, www.fertilitysociety.com.au/code-of-practice/.

Fertility Society of Australia & New Zealand 2020, Homepage, Fertility Society of Australia and New Zealand, www.fertilitysociety.com.au/.

Geller, S, Levy, S, Ashkeloni, S, Roeh, B, Sbiet, E & Avitsur, R 2021, 'Predictors of psychological distress in women with endometriosis: The role of multimorbidity, body image, and self-criticism', *International Journal of Environmental Research and Public Health,* vol. 18, no. 7, p. 3453.

Health Direct Australia 2022, 'Anti-inflammatory medicines (NSAIDs)', Health Direct, www.healthdirect.gov.au/anti-inflammatory-medicines.

Health Direct Australia 2023, 'Opioid medicines and pain', Health Direct, www.healthdirect.gov.au/opioids.

House of Wellness 2022, The House of Wellness, season 6, episode 25, Youtube, www.youtube.com/watch?v=SlfKqAm8RcI.

Jansson-Knodell, CL, King, KS, Larson, JJ, Van Dyke, CT, Murray, JA & Rubio-Tapia, A 2018, 'Gender-based differences in a population-based cohort with celiac disease: More alike than unalike', *Digestive Diseases and Sciences*, vol. 63, no. 1, pp. 184–92.

Jasinski, V, Voltolini Velho, R, Sehouli, J & Mechsner, S 2024, 'Cannabis use in endometriosis: the patients have their say — an online survey for German-speaking countries', *Archives of Gynecology and Obstetrics*.

Jean Hailes for Women's Health 2020, 'Endometriosis & natural therapies', Jean Hailes, www.jeanhailes.org.au/health-a-z/endometriosis/endometriosis-natural-therapies.

Jean Hailes for Women's Health 2023, 'Persistent pelvic pain', Jean Hailes, www.jeanhailes.org.au/health-a-z/persistent-pelvic-pain.

Julia Argyrou Endometriosis Centre at Epworth, Homepage, (JAECE), www.epworth.org.au/our-services/endometriosis-centre.

Kennedy, S, Bergqvist, A, Chapron, C, D'Hooghe, T, Dunselman, G, Greb, R, Hummelshoj, L, Prentice, A, Saridogan, E & ESHRE Special Interest Group for Endometriosis and Endometrium Guideline Development Group 2005, 'ESHRE guideline for the diagnosis and treatment of endometriosis', *Human Reproduction (Oxford, England)*, vol. 20, no. 10, pp. 2698–2704.

Kidspot 2024, 'Bindi Irwin's heartbreaking admission about having another baby: "She will be our one child"', *New York Post*, nypost.com/2024/08/30/entertainment/she-will-be-our-one-child-bindi-irwins-heartbreaking-admission-about-having-another-baby/.

Kvaskoff, M, Mu, F, Terry, KL, Harris, HR, Poole, EM, Farland, L & Missmer, SA 2015, 'Endometriosis: a high-risk population for major chronic diseases?' *Human reproduction Update*, vol. 21, no. 4, pp. 500–16.

Lang-Illievich, K, Klivinyi, C, Lasser, C, Brenna, CTA, Szilagyi, IS & Bornemann-Cimenti, H 2023, 'Palmitoylethanolamide in the treatment of chronic pain: A systematic review and meta-analysis of double-blind randomized controlled trials', *Nutrients*, vol. 15, no. 6.

Lee, J & Wheate, APN 2024, 'What is Ryeqo?', NewsGP, www1.racgp.org.au/newsgp/clinical/what-is-ryeqo.

Lim, MC & Pfaendler K 2017, 'Type and risk of cancer related to endometriosis: Ovarian cancer and beyond', BJOG, vol. 125, no. 1, p. 73.

Lima, RF, Maria da Silva Kotze, L, Kotze, LR, Chrisostomo, KR & Nisihara, R 2019, 'Gender-related differences in celiac patients at diagnosis', *Archives of Medical Research*, vol. 50, no. 7, pp. 437–41.

Liotta, M 2021, 'Delayed endometriosis diagnosis reduces chance of pregnancy by 33%', NewsGP, www1.racgp.org.au/newsgp/clinical/delayed-endometriosis-diagnosis-reduces-chance-of.

Mak, JN, Uzuner, C, Espada, M, Eathorn, A, Reid, S, Leonardi, M, Armour, M & Condous, GS 2024, 'Inter-observer reproducibility of the 2021 AAGL Endometriosis Classification', *The Australian & New Zealand Journal of Obstetrics & Gynaecology*, obgyn.onlinelibrary.wiley.com/doi/10.1111/ajo.13851.

Mardon, AK, Leake, HB, Szeto, K, Astill, T, Hilton, S, Moseley, GL & Chalmers, KJ 2022, 'Treatment recommendations for the management of persistent pelvic pain: a systematic review of international clinical practice guidelines', *BJOG: An International Journal of Obstetrics and Gynaecology*, vol. 129, no. 8, pp. 1248–60.

Margery-Muir, AA, Bundell, C, Nelson, D, Groth, DM & Wetherall, JD 2017, 'Gender balance in patients with systemic lupus erythematosus', *Autoimmunity Reviews*, vol. 16, no. 3, pp. 258–68.

Meints, SM & Edwards, RR 2018, 'Evaluating psychosocial contributions to chronic pain outcomes', *Progress in Neuro-Psychopharmacology & Biological Psychiatry*, vol. 87, no. Pt B, pp. 168–82.

Meresman, GF, Götte, M & Laschke, MW 2021, 'Plants as source of new therapies for endometriosis: a review of preclinical and clinical studies', *Human Reproduction Update,* vol. 27, no. 2, pp. 367–92.

Mortlock, S, Corona, RI, Kho, PF, Pharoah, P, Seo, J-H, Freedman, ML, Gayther, SA, Siedhoff, MT, Rogers, PAW, Leuchter, R, Walsh, CS, Cass, I, Karlan, BY, Rimel, BJ, Ovarian Cancer Association Consortium, International Endometriosis Genetics Consortium, Montgomery, GW, Lawrenson, K & Kar, SP 2022, 'A multi-level investigation of the genetic relationship between endometriosis and ovarian cancer histotypes', *Cell Reports Medicine*, vol. 3, no. 3, p. 100542.

National Institutes of Health 2024, 'Endometriosis types and ovarian cancer risk', NIH, nih.gov/news-events/nih-research-matters/endometriosis-types-ovarian-cancer-risk.

Naturopaths & Herbalists Association of Australia 2020, Homepage, NHAA, nhaa.org.au/.

Nezhat, F, Datta, MS, Hanson, V, Pejovic, T, Nezhat, C & Nezhat, C 2008, 'The relationship of endometriosis and ovarian malignancy: a review', *Fertility and Sterility*, vol. 90, no. 5, pp. 1559–70.

Oral, E 2022, 'Endometriosis and adenomyosis: Global perspectives across the lifespan', Springer Nature.

Osborne, NR & Davis, KD 2022, 'Sex and gender differences in pain', *International Review of Neurobiology*, vol. 164, pp. 277–307.

Ovarian Cancer Research Alliance 2022, 'Researchers discover genetic link between ovarian cancer subtypes and endometriosis', Ovarian Cancer Research Alliance, ocrahope.org/news/researchers-discover-genetic-link-between-ovarian-cancer-subtypes-and-endometriosis/.

Pehlivan, MJ, Sherman, KA, Wuthrich, V, Horn, M, Basson, M & Duckworth, T 2022, 'Body image and depression in endometriosis: Examining self-esteem and rumination as mediators', *Body Image*, vol. 43, pp. 463–73.

Pelvic Pain Foundation 2022, 'Painful sex – women', Pelvic Pain Foundation, www.pelvicpain.org.au/painful-sex-women/.

Pink Elephants Support Network n.d., 'Female fertility issues', Pink Elephants Support Network, www.pinkelephants.org.au/page/90/female-fertility-issues.

Rahmioglu, N, Mortlock, S, Ghiasi, Molller, PL, Stefansdorttir, L, Galarneau, G, et al. 2023, The genetic basis of endometriosis and comorbidity with other pain and inflammatory conditions', *Nature Genetics*, vol. 55, no. 3, pp. 423–36.

Rossi, MF, Tumminello, A, Marconi, M, Gualano, MR, Santoro, PE, Malorni, W & Moscato, U 2022, 'Sex and gender differences in migraines: a narrative review', *Neurological Sciences: Official Journal of the Italian Neurological Society and of the Italian Society of Clinical Neurophysiology*, vol. 43, no. 9, pp. 5729–34.

Royal Australian College of General Practitioners n.d., 'Management of persistent pelvic pain in girls and women', *Australian Family Physician*, vol. 44, no. 7.

Royal Women's Hospital n.d., 'Treating endometriosis', The Royal Women's Hospital, www.thewomens.org.au/health-information/periods/endometriosis/treating-endometriosis.

Rustgi, SD, Kayal, M & Shah, SC 2020, 'Sex-based differences in inflammatory bowel diseases: a review', *Therapeutic Advances in Gastroenterology*, vol. 13, p. 1756284820915043.

Samami, E, Shahhosseini, Z, Khani, S & Elyasi, FK 2023, 'Pain-focused psychological interventions in women with endometriosis: A systematic review', *Neuropsychopharmacol Rep*, vol. 43, no. 3, pp. 310–19.

Saunders, PTK, Whitaker, LHR, & Horne, AW 2024, 'Endometriosis: Improvements and challenges in diagnosis and symptom management', *Cell Reports Medicine*, vol. 5, no. 6, p. 101596.

Sayer-Jones, K & Sherman, KA 2023, '"My body...tends to betray me sometimes": a qualitative analysis of affective and perceptual body image in individuals living with endometriosis', *International Journal of Behavioral Medicine*, vol. 30, no. 4, pp. 543–54.

Schick, M, Germeyer, A, Böttcher, B, Hecht, S, Geiser, M, Rösner, S, Eckstein, M, Vomstein, K, Toth, B, Strowitzki, T, Wischmann, T & Ditzen, B 2022, 'Partners matter: The psychosocial well-being of couples when dealing with endometriosis', *Health and Quality of Life Outcomes,* vol. 20, no. 1, p. 86.

Seeley, M-C, Lau, DH, & Gallagher, C 2023, 'Postural orthostatic tachycardia syndrome: Diagnosis and management guide for nurses', *Nursing: Research and Reviews,* vol. 13, pp. 41–9.

Sempere, L, Bernabeu, P, Cameo, J, Gutiérrez, A, García, MG, García, MF, Aguas, M, Belén, O, Zapater, P, Jover, R, van-der Hofstadt, C & Ruiz-Cantero, MT 2023, 'Gender biases and diagnostic delay in inflammatory bowel disease: Multicenter observational study', *Inflammatory Bowel Diseases*, vol. 29, no. 12, pp. 1886–94.

Shah, R & Newcomb, DC 2018, 'Sex bias in asthma prevalence and pathogenesis', *Frontiers in Immunology*, vol. 9, p. 2997.

Singh, N & Sharma, R 2023, 'A conceptual view of endometriosis through an Ayurveda Perspective', *Journal of Ayurveda and Integrated Medical Sciences,* vol. 8, no. 3.

Sivananda Yoga Vedanta Centre 1996, *Practical Ayurveda: Find out who you are and what you need to bring balance to your life,* Dorling Kindersley.

Skinner M 2022, 'Can acupuncture reduce endometriosis pain?', Endometriosis Foundation of America, www.endofound.org/can-acupuncture-reduce-endometriosis-pain.

Slater, H, Jordan, JE, O'Sullivan, PB, Schütze, R, Goucke, R, Chua, J, Browne, A, Horgan, B, De Morgan, S & Briggs, AM 2022, '"Listen to me, learn from me": a priority setting partnership for shaping interdisciplinary pain training to strengthen chronic pain care', *Pain*, vol. 163, no. 11, pp. e1145–e1163.

Steinbuch, SC, Lüß, A-M, Eltrop S, Götte, M & Kiesel L 2024, 'Endometriosis-associated ovarian cancer: From molecular pathologies to clinical relevance, *Int J Mol Sci*, vol. 25, no. 8, p.4306.

Surrey, ES 2015, 'Endometriosis-related infertility: The role of the assisted reproductive technologies', *BioMed Research International*, vol. 2015, p. 482959.

Therapeutic Goods Administration n.d., What's on my medicine label?, TGA, www.tga.gov.au/products/medicines/find-information-about-medicine/whats-my-medicine-label#australian-register-of-therapeutic-goods-artg-number.

Therapeutic Goods Administration 2024, 'Medicinal cannabis hub', TGA, www.tga.gov.au/products/unapproved-therapeutic-goods/medicinal-cannabis-hub.

Therapeutic Goods Administration 2024, Ryeqo (Gedeon Richter Australia Pty Ltd), TGA, www.tga.gov.au/resources/prescription-medicines-registrations/ryeqo-gedeon-richter-australia-pty-ltd-0.

Thombre Kulkarni, M, Shafrir, A, Farland, LV, Terry, KL, Whitcomb, BW, Eliassen, AH, Bertone-Johnson, ER & Missmer, SA 2022, 'Association between laparoscopically confirmed endometriosis and risk of early natural menopause', JAMA Network Open, vol. 5, no. 1, p. e2144391.

University of Sydney n.d., 'History of cannabis', The University of Sydney, www.sydney.edu.au/lambert/medicinal-cannabis/history-of-cannabis.html#:~:text=The%20use%20of%20cannabis%20originated,father%20of%20Chinese%20medicine)%20pharmacopoeia.

van Vollenhoven, RF 2009, 'Sex differences in rheumatoid arthritis: more than meets the eye', BMC Medicine, vol. 7, no. 1, p. 12.

Vermeulen, N, Abrao, MS, Einarsson, JI, Horne, AW, Johnson, NP, Lee, TTM, Missmer, S, Petrozza, J, Tomassetti, C, Zondervan, KT, Grimbizis, G, De Wilde, RL, & International working group of AAGL, ESGE, ESHRE and WES 2021, 'Endometriosis classification, staging and reporting systems: A review on the road to a universally accepted endometriosis classification', Journal of Minimally Invasive Gynecology, vol. 28, no. 11, pp. 1822–48.

Victorian Assisted Reproductive Treatment Authority, n.d. 'Legislation and guidelines', VARTA, www.varta.org.au/regulation/legislation-and-guidelines.

Villnes Z 2023, 'Can acupuncture help endometriosis?', Medical News Today, www.medicalnewstoday.com/articles/acupuncture-for-endometriosis.

Volker, C & Mills, J 2022, 'Endometriosis and body image: Comparing people with and without endometriosis and exploring the relationship with pelvic pain', Body Image, vol. 43, pp. 518–22.

Watkins E n.d., Abstract and bio, Macquarie University, www.mq.edu.au/__data/assets/pdf_file/0019/1305424/Emma-Watkins-Abstract-Bio.pdf.

Weedmaps 2024, 'Marijuana is the "most effective" way for women with endometriosis to manage their symptoms, study finds', Weedmaps, weedmaps.com/news/2024/08/marijuana-is-the-most-effective-way-for-women-with-endometriosis-to-manage-their-symptoms-study-finds/.

Wood R n.d., 'A potted history of the Endometriosis Association Victoria', Endometriosis.org, endometriosis.org/news/support-awareness/endometriosis-association-victoria-celebrates-21-years/.

Zhong, C, Gao, L, Shu, L, Hou, Z, Cai, L, Huang, J, Liu, J & Mao, Y 2021, 'Analysis of IVF/ICSI outcomes in endometriosis patients with recurrent implantation failure: Influence on cumulative live birth rate', *Frontiers in Endocrinology (Lausanne)*, www.frontiersin.org/journals/endocrinology/articles/10.3389/fendo.2021.640288/full. [epub]

Part IV: Try it out

Amini, M, Zayeri, F & Salehi, M 2021, 'Trend analysis of cardiovascular disease mortality, incidence, and mortality-to-incidence ratio: results from global burden of disease study 2017', BMC Public Health, vol. 21, no. 401.

Arab, A, Karimi, E, Vingrys, K, Kelishadi, MR, Mehrabani, S & Askari, G 2022, 'Food groups and nutrients consumption and risk of endometriosis: a systematic review and meta-analysis of observational studies', *Nutrition Journal*, vol. 21, no. 1, p. 58.

Australian Commission on Safety and Quality Health Care n.d., 'Australian Charter of Healthcare Rights', Australian Commission on Safety and Quality Health Care, www.safetyandquality.gov.au/our-work/partnering-consumers/australian-charter-healthcare-rights.

Barnard, ND, Holtz, DN, Schmidt, N, Kolipaka, S, Hata, E, Sutton, M, Znayenko-Miller, T, Hazen, ND, Cobb, C & Kahleova, H 2023, 'Nutrition in the prevention and treatment of endometriosis: A review', *Frontiers in Nutrition*, vol. 10, p. 1089891.

Better Health n.d., 'Soybeans and soy foods', Better Health, www.betterhealth.vic.gov.au/health/healthyliving/soybeans.

Brouns, F, Van Haaps, A, Keszthelyi, D, Venema, K, Bongers, M, Maas, J & Mijatovic, V 2023, 'Diet associations in endometriosis: a critical narrative assessment with special reference to gluten', *Frontiers in Nutrition*, vol. 10, p. 1166929.

Cai, X, Liu, M, Zhang, B, Zhao, S-J & Jiang, S-W,2021, 'Phytoestrogens for the management of endometriosis: Findings and issues', *Pharmaceuticals (Basel, Switzerland)*, vol. 14, no. 6, p. 569.

Cervoni, B 2023, 'How to follow an endometriosis diet', Verywell Health, www.verywellhealth.com/endometriosis-diet-7105372.

Cleveland Clinic 2022, 'The best and worst foods for an anti-inflammatory endometriosis diet', Cleveland Clinic, health.clevelandclinic.org/endometriosis-diet.

Endometriosis Foundation of America 2018, 'Check, Please! The 10 foods endo women should avoid', Endometriosis Foundation of America, www.endofound.org/10-foods-endo-women-should-avoid.

Endo Zone n.d., 'Low FODMAP diet', EndoZone, www.endozone.com.au/treatment/121.

Evans, S, Villegas, V, Dowding, C, Druitt, M, O'Hara, R & Mikocka-Walus, A 2022, 'Treatment use and satisfaction in Australian women with endometriosis: a mixed-methods study', *Internal Medicine Journal*, vol. 52, no. 12, pp. 2096–2106.

Fody n.d., 'The foods you should eat (and avoid) with endometriosis', FODY, www.fodyfoods.com/blogs/in-the-news/if-you-suffer-from-endometriosis-these-are-the-foods-you-should-eat-and-avoid.

Fowke, JH, Longcope, C, Hebert, JR 2000, 'Brassica vegetable consumption shifts estrogen metabolism in healthy menopausal women', *Cancer Epidemiology, Biomarkers and Prevention*, vol. 9, no. 8, pp. 773–9.

Fujioka, N, Ransom, BW, Carmella, SG, Upadhyaya, P, Lindgren, BR, Roper-Batker A, et al., 'Harnessing the power of cruciferous vegetables: Developing a biomarker for Brassica vegetable consumption using urinary 3,3'-diindolylmethane', *Cancer Prevention Research*, vol. 9, no. 10, pp 788–93.

Goltsman, D, Li, Z, Bruce, E, Darton, A, Thornbury, K, Maitz, PKM & Kennedy, P 2015, 'Too hot to handle? Hot water bottle injuries in Sydney, Australia', *Burns: Journal of the International Society for Burn Injuries*, vol. 41, no. 4, pp. 770–77.

Greger, M, Stone, G 2016, *How not to die*, Macmillan.

Harris, HR, Chavarro, JE, Malspeis, S, Willett, WC & Missmer, SA 2013, 'Dairy-food, calcium, magnesium, and vitamin D intake and endometriosis: a prospective cohort study', *American Journal of Epidemiology*, vol. 177, no. 5, pp. 420–30.

Harris, HR, Eke, AC, Chavarro, JE, Missmer, SA n.d., 'Fruit and vegetable consumption and risk of endometriosis', Human Reproduction, vol. 33, no. 4, pp. 715–27.

Health Outcomes n.d., 'The endometriosis health profile (EHP)', Health Outcomes, innovation.ox.ac.uk/outcome-measures/endometriosis-health-profile-ehp/.

Itsines K 2024, 'Kayla Itsine's endometriosis-friendly workout', Women's Health, womenshealth.com.au/kayla-itsines-endometriosis-friendly-workout/.

Itsines K 2024, 'Try gentle strength: An endometriosis-friendly workout from Kayla Itsines', Sweat, https://sweat.com/blogs/wellbeing/endometriosis-awareness-month-workout.

Joy R 2023, 'What to know about cold water therapy', Healthline, www.healthline.com/health/cold-water-therapy.

Mardon, AK, Leake, HB, Hayles, C, Henry, ML, Neumann, PB, Moseley, GL & Chalmers, KJ 2023, 'The efficacy of self-management strategies for females with endometriosis: A systematic review', *Reproductive Sciences (Thousand Oaks, Calif.)*, vol. 30, no. 2, pp. 390–407.

Miserandino, C 2013, 'The spoon theory written by Christine Miserandino', But You Dont Look Sick?, butyoudontlooksick.com/articles/written-by-christine/the-spoon-theory/.

Monash University, 'Low FODMAP diet', Monash University, www.monashfodmap.com/.

Perillo S, 'Cold water swimming: Do the benefits really outweigh the risks', Herald Sun, www.heraldsun.com.au/news/victoria/cold-water-swimming-do-the-benefits-really-outweigh-the-risks/news-story/645d5cba9e51378074f5e712d598e5bd.

Reynolds, J 2024, 'Ice baths to treat endometriosis pain?', iCoolsport, icoolsport.com/blogs/therapy/ice-baths-to-treat-endometriosis-pain.

Sherwood, RA, Rocks, BF, Stewart, A & Saxton, RS 1986, 'Magnesium and the premenstrual syndrome', *Annals of Clinical Biochemistry*, vol. 23, no. 6, pp. 667–70.

Sidharthan, C 2024, 'Researchers reveal why a diet rich in magnesium is so important for your health', News Medical, www.news-medical.net/news/20240815/Researchers-reveal-why-a-diet-rich-in-magnesium-is-so-important-for-your-health.aspx.

Twinings n.d., 'Tea and caffeine', Twinings, twinings.com.au/blogs/all-about-tea/tea-and-caffeine.

Ty, N 2023, 'Hot water bottle horror: Melbourne woman suffers "traumatic" injuries from common household item', 9News, www.9news.com.au/national/melbourne-woman-suffers-traumatic-injuries-from-hot-water-bottle/7c613006-5510-4da2-915b-2e7b07fce503.

van Haaps, AP, Wijbers, JV, Schreurs, AMF, Vlek, S, Tuynman, J, De Bie, B, de Vogel, AL, can Wely, M, Mijatovic, V 2023, 'The effect of dietary interventions on pain and quality of life in women diagnosed with endometriosis: a prospective study with control group', *Human Reproduction,* vol. 38, no. 12, pp. 2433–46.

World Health Organization 2024, 'Self-care for health and well-being', WHO, www.who.int/health-topics/self-care.

Yalçın Bahat, P, Ayhan, I, Üreyen Özdemir, E, İnceboz, Ü & Oral, E 2022, 'Dietary supplements for treatment of endometriosis: A review', *Acta Bio-Medica*, vol. 93, no. 1, p. e2022159.

Part V: Take it on

Australian Centre for Accelerating Diabetes Innovations 2023, 'Diabetes in Australia', ACADI, www.aph.gov.au/DocumentStore.ashx?id=da78917e-e885-49a0-9775-143b071ca756&subId=747694.

Australian Human Rights Commission n.d., Homepage, Australian Human Rights Commission, defence.humanrights.gov.au/.

Australian Institute of Health and Welfare 2023, 'Endometriosis', AIHW, www.aihw.gov.au/reports/chronic-disease/endometriosis-in-australia/contents/summary.

Bourdon, M, Maignien, C, Giraudet, G, Estrade, JP, Indersie, E, Solignac, C, Arbo, E, Roman, H, Chapron, C, Santulli, P 2024, 'Investigating the medical journey of endometriosis-affected women: Results from a cross-sectional web-based survey (EndoVie) on 1,557 French women', *Journal of Gynecology Obstetrics and Human Reproduction*, 53(2):102708, doi:10.1016/j.jogoh.2023.102708.

Brunak, S, Wetergaard, D & Krabbe, C 2019, 'Study: Across diseases, women are diagnosed later than men', Novo Nordisk Foundation Center for Protein Research, www.cpr.ku.dk/cpr-news/2019/study-across-diseases-women-are-diagnosed-later-than-men/.

Cameron, L, Mikocka-Walus, A, Sciberras, E, Druitt, M, Stanley, K & Evans, S 2024, 'Menstrual pain in Australian adolescent girls and its impact on regular activities: a population-based cohort analysis based on Longitudinal Study of Australian Children survey data', *The Medical Journal of Australia*, vol. 220, no. 9, pp. 466–71.

Davey, M 2022, '"No one would believe me": Labor launches women's health council to tackle medical misogyny', The Guardian, www.theguardian .com/australia-news/2022/dec/08/labor-launches-national-womens-health-advisory-council-to-tackle-medical-misogyny.

Department of Health and Aged Care, 2024, '2 out of 3 women experience discrimination in healthcare', Australian Government, www.health.gov .au/ministers/the-hon-ged-kearney-mp/media/2-out-of-3-women-experience-discrimination-in-healthcare-0#:~:text=The%20Hon%20 Ged%20Kearney%20MP,-Assistant%20Minister%20for&text=Two%20 out%20of%20three%20women,relation%20to%20diagnosis%20 and%20treatment.

Department of Health and Aged Care 2024, 'End gender bias survey results – summary report', Australian Government, www.health.gov .au/womens-health-advisory-council/resources/publications/ endgenderbias-survey-results-summary-report?language=en.

Department of Health and Aged Care 2024, 'National Women's Health Advisory Council', Australian Government, www.health.gov.au/womens-health-advisory-council.

Department of Health and Aged Care 2024, 'Reforming the health system to improve sexual and reproductive care', Australian Government, www.health.gov.au/ministers/the-hon-ged-kearney-mp/media/reforming-the-health-system-to-improve-sexual-and-reproductive-care.

Endometriosis.org n.d., Homepage, Endometriosis.org, endometriosis.org/#google_vignette.

Department of Social Services 2023, 'Growing Up in Australia: The Longitudinal Study of Australian Children (LSAC)', Australian Government, www.dss.gov.au/about-the-department/longitudinal-studies/growing-up-in-australia-lsac-longitudinal-study-of-australian-children-overview.

Endometriosis WA 2022, 'LGBTQIA+ and Endo', Endometriosis WA, www.endometriosiswa.org.au/im-seeking-support/endometriosis-and-gender-diversity/.

Fair Work Commission 2009, 'Unreasonable refusal of a support person', Australian Government, www.fwc.gov.au/unreasonable-refusal-support-person.

Ghin, P, Adamovic, M & Ainsworth, S 2023, 'Disclosing illness at work: A survey of leaders living and working with chronic illness', The University of Melbourne, fbe.unimelb.edu.au/__data/assets/pdf_file/0007/4639318/Disclosing_Illness_at_Work_Ghin_Ainsworth.pdf.

Heaney, C 2024, 'GPs urged to ask about period pain early', NewsGP, www1.racgp.org.au/newsgp/clinical/gps-urged-to-screen-for-period-pain-early.

Humphreys, L 2023, 'Take care with hot water bottles this winter', Alfred Health, www.alfredhealth.org.au/news/take-care-with-hot-water-bottles-this-winter/.

Jean Hailes for Women's Health n.d., 'First Nations resources', Jean Hailes for Women's Health, www.jeanhailes.org.au/resources/aboriginal-and-torres-strait-islander-resources.

Lang, K 2022, 'Endometriosis: Why is there so little research?', Medical News Today, www.medicalnewstoday.com/articles/endometriosis-why-is-there-so-little-research.

LGBTIQ+ Health Australia n.d., Homepage, LGBTIQ+ Health Australia, www.lgbtiqhealth.org.au/.

Moradi, M, Parker, M, Sneddon, A, Lopez, V & Ellwood, D 2014, 'Impact of endometriosis on women's lives: a qualitative study', *BMC Women's Health*, vol. 14, no. 1, p. 123.

Moradi, M, Parker, M, Sneddon, A, Lopez, V & Ellwood, D 2019, 'The Endometriosis Impact Questionnaire (EIQ): a tool to measure the long-term impact of endometriosis on different aspects of women's lives', *BMC Women's Health*, vol. 19, no. 1, p. 64.

Müller, L 2023, 'FemXX's LGBTQIA+ Endo Resource Hub', FemXX Health, www.femxx.health/post/lgbtqia.

Munro, C & Grover, SR 2024, 'Ending the neglect of menstrual pain in adolescents is the key to improving outcomes for people with persistent pelvic pain', *The Medical Journal of Australia*, vol. 220, no. 9, pp. 459–60.

Murdoch Children's Research Institute n.d., LongSTEPPP Project, Murdoch Children's Research Institute, www.mcri.edu.au/research/projects/longsteppp.

Nancy's Nook 2021, 'LGBTQIA+ resources', NancysNookEndo, nancysnookendo.com/lgbtqia-resources/.

National Aboriginal Community Controlled Health Organisation (NACCHO) n.d., Homepage, NACCHO, www.naccho.org.au/.

New South Wales Consolidated Acts n.d., 'Work Health and Safety Act 2011 - Sect 28', New South Wales Consolidated Acts, classic.austlii.edu.au/au/legis/nsw/consol_act/whasa2011218/s28.html.

Nnoaham, KE, Hummelshoj, L, Webster, P & D'Hooghe, T 2011, 'Impact of endometriosis on quality of life and work productivity: A multicenter study across ten countries', *Fertility and Sterility*, Australian Institute of Health and Welfare, vol. 96, no. 2, pp. 366–73.

Pelvic Pain Foundation n.d., PPEP Talk: Periods, pain and endometriosis education for students in year 9 and above, Pelvic Pain Foundation, www.pelvicpain.org.au/ppep-talk-schools-program/.

RACGP 2023, 'Health of the nation', RACGP, www.racgp.org.au/general-practice-health-of-the-nation-2023.

RACGP 2024, 'RACGP gender equity IWD 2024', RACGP, www.racgp.org.au/gp-news/media-releases/2024-media-releases/march-2024/racgp-calls-for-equity-for-australia-s-women-gps-o.

Rowlands, I, Mishra, G & Abbott, J 2022, 'Endo can end women's careers and stall their education', The University of Queensland, public-health.uq.edu.au/article/2022/03/endometriosis-can-end-women%E2%80%99s-careers-and-stall-their-education-%E2%80%99everyone%E2%80%99s-business.

Safe Work Australia 2019, 'Supporting workers with endometriosis in the workplace', Safe Work Australia, www.safeworkaustralia.gov.au/doc/supporting-workers-endometriosis-workplace.

Slawson, N 2019, '"Women have been woefully neglected": Does medical science have a gender problem?', The Guardian, www.theguardian.com/education/2019/dec/18/women-have-been-woefully-neglected-does-medical-science-have-a-gender-problem.

Sperschneider, ML, Hengartner, MP, Kohl-Schwartz, A, Geraedts, K, Rauchfuss, M, Woelfler, MM, Haeberlin, F, von Orelli, S, Eberhard, M, Maurer, F, Imthurn, B, Imesch, P & Leeners, B 2019, 'Does endometriosis affect professional life? A matched case-control study in Switzerland, Germany and Austria', BMJ Open, vol. 9, no. 1, p. e019570.

Thorne Harbour Health, Homepage, Thorne Harbour Health, thorneharbour.org/.

WorkSafe Victoria n.d., 'Occupational health and safety - your legal duties', WorkSafe Victoria, www.worksafe.vic.gov.au/occupational-health-and-safety-your-legal-duties.

World Health Organization n.d., 'Years of healthy life lost due to disability (YLD)', WHO, www.who.int/data/gho/indicator-metadata-registry/imr-details/160.

Part VI: Take action

Brodtmann G, '#1in10 women have endometriosis', Youtube, www.youtube.com/watch?v=IVXw0kjxZd4.

Department of Health 2018, 'National action plan for endometriosis', Australian Government, www.health.gov.au/sites/default/files/national-action-plan-for-endometriosis.pdf.

Endometriosis.org, n.d., 'World Endometriosis Organisations, Endometriosis.org, endometriosis.org/support/world-endometriosis-organisations-weo/.

NECST Network n.d., 'The NECST Registry', UNSW Sydney, www.unsw.edu.au/research/necstnetwork/registry.

Private Healthcare Australia 2023, 'Australians sign up to private health insurance in record numbers', Private Healthcare Australia, privatehealthcareaustralia.org.au/australians-sign-up-to-private-health-insurance-in-record-numbers/.

World Endometriosis Society n.d., 'World congress on endometriosis 2025' WCE2025, www.wce2025.com.au/org-committee.

World Health Organization 2023, 'Endometriosis', WHO, www.who.int/news-room/fact-sheets/detail/endometriosis.

Index

AAGL *see* American Association of Gynecologic Laparoscopists (AAGL)

Abbott, Jason 53, 260–261, 269, 276

abdominal and pelvic pain, causes of 20
  anaemia 23–24
  fatigue or low energy 22–23
  fibroids 22
  inflammatory bowel disease 21
  interstitial cystitis 21
  mesenteric adenitis 21–22
  myalgic encephalomyelitis 23
  pelvic inflammatory disease 22
  polycystic ovarian syndrome (PCOS) 22
  small intestinal bacterial overgrowth (SIBO) 20–21
  urinary tract infections 21

abdominal exercises, protecting with 179

abdominal hysterectomy 85

Aboriginal and Torres Strait Islanders 207, 240

abortion 12

About Bloody Time 29, 61, 211–212

acupuncture 122, 287

adenomyosis 8, 12, 91, 102, 103, 151
  resources for 282

adhesions 4, 6, 91, 103, 126

adolescent girls, with endometriosis 202–204

AFCA *see* Australian Financial Complaints Authority (AFCA)

AGES *see* Australasian Gynaecological Endoscopy and Surgery Society (AGES)

agni 78

Ainsworth, Anna 271

Ainsworth, Simon 271

ALA *see* alpha-linolenic acid (ALA)

allied health practitioners 114
  pelvic physiotherapy 115–116
alpha-linolenic acid (ALA) 162
ALSWH *see* Australian
  Longitudinal Study
  on Women+'s Health
  (ALSWH)
American Association
  of Gynecologic
  Laparoscopists (AAGL) 9
AMH *see* anti-Mullerian
  hormone (AMH)
anaemia 23–24
analgesics 66
Andrew, Rachel 52–53, 118–122
anti-inflammatory diet 161–162
anti-Mullerian hormone
  (AMH) 93
antioxidants and gut health
  164–165
ART *see* assisted reproductive
  technology (ART)
ashwagandha 78
asking, art of 224
aspirin 66
assisted reproductive technology
  (ART) 71
Australasian Gynaecological
  Endoscopy and Surgery
  Society (AGES) 12
Australian Charter of Health
  Care Rights 152
Australian Financial Complaints
  Authority (AFCA) 209
Australian Longitudinal Study
  on Women+'s Health
  (ALSWH) 8

Australian workplace laws
  223–224
autonomy for patients 153
awareness of endometriosis
  249–250
Ayurvedic herbal therapies
  77–78

backwards menstruation *see*
  retrograde menstruation
Balasana 176
barley 164
Bayer 35
beans 157
bedside evaluation 60
belly button 82
belly, endo 7
berries 157
beverages 158
biopsychosocial approaches
  107–108
bleeding between menstrual
  periods 6
bloating, xvii 7, 157, 265, 286
blood clots 35, 68–70
The Blue Zones Solution
  (Dalai Lama and Dan
  Buettner) 157
body image 7, 132
boswellia 78
Brassica genus 155
bridge pose (Setu Bandhasana)
  178
Brodtmann, Gai 262, 268
Brown, Kylie 264
Bush, Deborah 270
butterfly stretch 178

caffeine 162
CALD backgrounds *see* culturally and linguistically diverse (CALD) backgrounds
cannabidiol (CBD) 72
care team and plan 41
  general practitioner management plan 42
  general practitioner mental health treatment plan 42–43
  team care arrangements 42
Cartwright, Lexie 29
cat-cow stretch 176–177
causes of endometriosis 13
CBD *see* cannabidiol (CBD)
celecoxib 66
chamomile 77
Chesters, Lisa 263
chest pain 7
chia seeds 162
child's pose (Balasana) 176
Chinese herbal medicine 77
chocolate cysts *see* ovarian endometriomas
chronic fatigue syndrome *see* myalgic encephalomyelitis
chronic pelvic pain syndrome, defined 17
clear cell carcinoma 26
codeine 66
cold shower at home 194
cold water therapy 192
  benefits of 192–193
  for endometriosis research at the University of Adelaide 194–195
  practice 193–194

safety precautions 195
Colgrave, Eliza 165–168
contraception 70, 71, 92
couples counselling 145–146
COVID-19 pandemic 141, 189, 222, 255
COX-2 inhibitors 66
cramps, menstrual 4–5, 196
Crohn's disease 21
cruciferous vegetables 157
culturally and linguistically diverse (CALD) backgrounds 250
cupping 124
curcumin 78
cyclical *vs.* non-cyclical periods 4–5
cysteine 165
cystic ovarian endometriosis 10

dads as endo supporters 141–142
Daily Dozen 157–158
daily life and responsibilities 147–148
dairy products 155
dandelion 77
dark chocolate 164
deep endometriosis 10
deep infiltrating endometriosis (DIE) 4
  DIE I 10
  DIE II 10
DHA *see* docosahexaenoic acid (DHA)
dhatus 78
diagnosis of endometriosis 12, 30–31

diclofenac 66
DIE *see* deep infiltrating
endometriosis (DIE)
diet and exercise, balancing
165–168
diet and nutrition 155–157
adapting to individual
health needs
158–159
anti-inflammatory diet
161–162
antioxidants and gut health
164–165
Daily Dozen 157–158
fermented foods, benefits
of 165
FODMAP diet 158, 159
high FODMAP
foods 160
low-FODMAP foods
159–160
gut microbiota 163
Heal. Nourish. Support.
Balance. 169
magnesium 169–170
supplements 169
omega 3 fatty acids 162
soy 162–163
digestive and gastrointestinal
symptoms of
endometriosis 7
digestive system 20, 156,
161, 164
discrimination against women+
232–233
docosahexaenoic acid
(DHA) 162

doctors for endometriosis 39
general practitioners (GPs)
40–41, 44
management plan 42
mental health treatment plan
42–43
gynaecologist 47–49
team care arrangements 42
dong quai 77
donor eggs 93–94
doshas 78
douching 12
doxylamine 66
Dr. Greger's Daily Dozen app 157
dry needling 124
enhanced blood flow and
healing 125
muscle pain relief,
targeted 124
muscle tension, reduction
of 125
neuromuscular reset 125
Dymadon 66
dysbiosis 163
dyschezia 30
dysmenorrhoea 30
dyspareunia 6, 30
dysuria 30

ECS *see* endocannabinoid
system (ECS)
Eden Foundation 271
educational resources 145
education and guidelines
for health, allied and
integrative practitioners
284–285

education for young girls and
women+ 283
eggs
donor 93–94
freezing 93
retrieval 95, 98, 100
eicosapentaenoic acid (EPA) 162
Eka Pada Rajakapotasana 178
embryo culture 95
embryo transfer 95
emotional issues 12
emotional support 126,
128–129
employee rights and workplace
flexibility in Australia
216–217
employer obligations 226
#EndGenderBias survey
233–234
endocannabinoid system (ECS)
72
endocrine disruptors 14–15
EndoFound Classification 9–10
endometrioid carcinoma 26
Endometriosis Management Plan
(Endo-MP) 250
Endo-MP see Endometriosis
Management Plan
(Endo-MP)
Endone 67
EndoZone 52, 62, 118, 145,
224, 263, 279
energy, lack of 22–23
environmental factors affecting
hormones 14–15
EPA see eicosapentaenoic acid
(EPA)
epigenetic process 14

ESHRE see European Society of
Human Reproduction and
Embryology (ESHRE)
estradiol 13
estrogen 14, 67, 68, 156
European Society of Human
Reproduction and
Embryology (ESHRE) 69
examinations and tests for
endometriosis 51
Imagendo project 55
medical imaging 54
pelvic examination 53–54
physical exam, preparing for
52–53
symptoms and testing 58
tests at the gyno 60–62
ultrasound 54–55
exercises 128, 158, 165–168,
173, 174, 290–291
abdominal 179
and stretches
bridge pose 178
butterfly stretch 178
cat-cow stretch 176–177
child's pose 176
hip flexor stretch 177–178
knee-to-chest stretch 177
pelvic tilts 177
pigeon pose 178
reclined bound angle
pose 177
seated forward bend 177

Faculty of Pain Medicine
of the Australian and
New Zealand College of
Anaesthetists 84

Index **321**

Fair Work Act 2009 215, 216, 224
Fair Work Ombudsman 215
family planning
  clinics 285
  endometriosis and its impact on 146
fatigue and Spoon Theory 188–190
fatigue/low energy 22–23
fats, healthy 162
fatty fish 162
Federal Department of Health and Aged Care 72
fermentable oligosaccharides, disaccharides, monosaccharides and polyols (FODMAP) diet *see* FODMAP diet
fermented foods, benefits of 165
fertility *see also* infertility; IVF process
  endo impacting 90–92, 95–97
  expectations from fertility specialist 92–93
  treatment options 93
    donor eggs 93–94
    freezing eggs 93
Fertility Society of Australia and New Zealand 92, 285
fibroids 22
financial stress resources 286
flaxseeds 158, 162
Flint, Nicolle 268
FODMAP diet 158, 159, 286–287
  high FODMAP foods 160
  low-FODMAP foods 159–160

follicle-stimulating hormone (FSH) 93
fruits 155, 157
FSH *see* follicle-stimulating hormone (FSH)
Fung, Anita 264
future of endo research and policy 259
  global endo efforts 267
    World Congress on Endometriosis 2025 Sydney 269
    World Endometriosis Organisations (WEO) 269–270
    World Endometriosis Society (WES) 269
  multi-disciplinary support for people with endometriosis 260–261
  National Action Plan on Endometriosis 263
  National Endometriosis Clinical Scientific Trials Registry 259–260
  Parliamentary Friends of Endometriosis Awareness 262–263
  pelvic pain clinics, endometriosis and 263–264
  philanthropy, gift of 270
    Eden Foundation 271
    Lambert Initiative 271
    Wilson Foundation 270

GABA *see* gamma-aminobutyric acid (GABA)
Gadd, Lisa 174

Gadd's endometriosis
stretches to attain
'living health' 176
bridge pose 178
butterfly stretch 178
cat-cow stretch 176–177
child's pose 176
hip flexor stretch
177–178
knee-to-chest stretch 177
pelvic tilts 177
pigeon pose 178
reclined bound angle
pose 177
seated forward bend 177
gamma-aminobutyric acid
(GABA) 170
gastrointestinal (GI) issues
7–8, 161
gendernomics in women+'s
health 207
under-and unemployment,
endo's impact on
209–210
UTERUSopia 208
UTERUSurper 208–209
general practitioners (GPs)
39–41
gender pay gap 237
management plan 42
mental health treatment plan
42–43
genetic and molecular links 26
genetics and gastrointestinal
issues 7–8
GI issues *see* gastrointestinal (GI)
issues
ginger 77

gingko biloba 77
ginseng 77
girls, adolescent, with
endometriosis
202–204
global endo efforts 267
World Congress on
Endometriosis 2025
Sydney 269
World Endometriosis
Organisations (WEO)
269–270
World Endometriosis Society
(WES) 269
Grover, Sonia 84
gluten-free coeliac 166
GnRH agonists 70
GnRH antagonists 70–71
GPs *see* general practitioners
(GPs)
Grace, Georgia 147
GRACE research group *see*
Gynaecological Research
and Clinical Evaluation
(GRACE) research
group
greens 158
grey matter 19, 20
gut health, antioxidants and
164–165
gut microbiota and
endometriosis 163
Gynaecological Research and
Clinical Evaluation
(GRACE) research group
260
gynaecologist for endometriosis
47–49

headaches 7
Heal. Nourish. Support.
  Balance. 169
  magnesium 169–170
  supplements 169
healthy fats 162
Healy, David 139
heat therapy 196
  usage considerations 196
heavy menstrual bleeding 5–6,
  23, 24, 35. 40, 281
herbal medicines, Chinese 77
herbs and spices 158, 287
high-grade serous carcinoma 26
hip flexor stretch 177–178
holistic approach 124, 280
holistic care 116–118
hormone-releasing intrauterine
  device 91
hormones, environmental factors
  affecting 14–15
hormone treatments 12, 40,
  67–69, 82, 174
  GnRH agonists 70
  GnRH antagonists
    70–71
  medicinal cannabis
    71–72
  oral contraceptive pill
    (OCP) 69
  oral progestins 70
  progesterone-like
    hormones 70
How Not to Die (Michael Greger
  and Gene Stone) 157
Hunt, Greg 262, 268
hysterectomy 12, 85

hysterosalpingo-contrast-
  ultrasonography
  (HyCoSy) 93

IBS see irritable bowel
  syndrome (IBS)
ibuprofen 66
Imagendo project 55
Increasing Awareness of
  Endometriosis Amongst
  Priority Populations
  264
Indian Ayurvedic herbal
  therapies 77–78
infertility 285 see also fertility;
  IVF process
  treatment options for,
    97–98
inflammation 3, 4, 6, 90, 121,
  123, 124, 159, 162, 163,
  169, 192
  chronic 22, 161, 165
  and nerves 18–19
inflammatory bowel disease 21
informed decision-making, xxii
  153
insemination and fertilisation 95
integrative health 131
integrative medicine 152
intersectionality and inclusion in
  care 239
  Aboriginal and Torres Strait
    Islanders 240
  awareness of endometriosis
    249–250
  LGBTQIA+ 250–251
interstitial cystitis 21

intimacy
  beyond sexuality 147
  sex and 147, 291
intimate relationships,
    endometriosis and its
    impact on 142–143
intrauterine devices (IUDs) 91,
    234, 251
irregular periods 5–6
irritable bowel syndrome
    (IBS) 7
Irwin, Bindi 90
Itsines, Kayla 264
IUDs see intrauterine devices
    (IUDs)
IVF process 71, 94
  costs 94
  next steps in 95

JAECE see Julia Argyrou
    Endometriosis Centre
    at Epworth (JAECE)
James, Akaiti 116–118
Jean Hailes Foundation for
    Women's Health 18, 21,
    240, 273, 274, 280
joints 6
Julia Argyrou Endometriosis
    Centre at Epworth
    (JAECE) 270, 280
justice in healthcare\ 153

Kapurubandara, Supruni 53
Kearney, Ged 233, 263, 264, 268
kefir 165
knee-to-chest stretch 177
kombucha 165

lacto-fermented vegetables 165
Lambert, Barry 271
Lambert, Joy 271
Lambert Initiative 271
laparoscopic hysterectomy 85
laparoscopic surgery, xviii 34,
    81–85
LARCs see long-acting reversible
    contraceptives (LARCs)
leg pain 6–7
leiomyoma see fibroids
lemon balm 77
Lemsip 66
lesions 3–4, 6–7, 10, 19, 91
levels of endometriosis 8–10
LGBTIQA+ community
    250–251, 287–288
LH see luteinising hormone
    (LH)
lifestyle and self-care 151–154
Living Health Group 174
Long, Barbara 262
long-acting reversible
    contraceptives
    (LARCs) 234
long-chain omega-3 fatty
    acids 155
Longitudinal Study of Australian
    Children (LSAC) 203
Longitudinal Study of
    Teenagers with
    Endometriosis, Period and
    Pelvic Pain (LongSTEPPP)
    205, 263
LSAC see Longitudinal Study
    of Australian Children
    (LSAC)

Index   325

Lucky, Tarana 48–49,
   60–62, 82
luteinising hormone (LH) 93
lymphatic drainage 123

magnesium 169–170
magnetic resonance imaging
   (MRI) technology, xviii 19,
   54, 55, 62, 233
magnetic resonance spectroscopy
   19
malas 78
Marino, Nola 263
massage therapy for
   endometriosis 125–126
Mazza, Danielle 44–46, 68
medical costs and
   rebates 289
medical imaging 54
medical misogyny 208, 231,
   232, 289
   end gender bias survey
      233–234
   general practitioner (GP)
      gender pay gap 237
   medical world excluding
      and ignoring women+
      232–233
   research funding, bias in
      237–238
Medicare 267
Medicare Benefits Schedule item
   12312, 232
medicinal cannabis 71–72, 287
medicinal herbs 77
melatonin 169
meloxicam 66

menopause 6, 22, 70, 90, 103,
   232, 261
menstrual bleeding, heavy 5–6,
   23, 24, 35, 40, 281
menstrual cramps 4–5, 196
menstrual cycle 3, 5, 9, 11, 13,
   31, 68, 90, 91, 143
menstrual periods 4, 85, 89,
   90, 103
   bleeding between 6
   cyclical vs. non-cyclical 4–5
   heavy 22
   irregular 5–6
   normal 5
   painful 5, 8, 9,
      12, 30, 35, 69, 142,
      203–205, 207
   progression 5
   severity 4
   timing and duration 4
menstruation 3, 5, 7,
   9, 21, 70, 205,
   239, 251
   painful 125
   retrograde 13, 170
mental health and wellbeing
   national support numbers
      288–289
Mersyndol 66
mesenteric adenitis 21–22
migraines 7, 40, 170
mind-body practices 128
Mishra, Gita 8, 214, 269
Montgomery, Grant 8
Mooney, Samantha 97–98
Moradi, Maryam 249–250
Morrison, Jenny 263

Morrison, Scott 263
most bothersome symptom 31
MRI technology *see* magnetic
  resonance imaging (MRI)
  technology
multidisciplinary care 107,
  260–261
  acupuncture 122
  allied health practitioners 114
  pelvic physiotherapy
    115–116
  biopsychosocial approaches
    107–108
  body image 132
  dry needling for endometriosis
    124
  enhanced blood flow and
    healing 125
  muscle pain relief,
    targeted 124
  muscle tension, reduction
    of 125
  neuromuscular reset 125
  emotional support 128–129
  holistic care 116–118
  integrative health 131
  massage therapy 125–127
  mind-body practices 128
  osteopathy for
    endometriosis 123
  cupping 124
  holistic approach 124
  improved circulation and
    lymphatic drainage 123
  pain relief 123
  pelvic health 123
  stress reduction 123

pacing activities 128
patients' varied needs,
  supporting 110–114
physical activity and
  exercise 127
physiotherapy 118–122
psychological support 127
sleep hygiene 128
stress management 128
muscle pain relief, targeted 124
muscle tension, reduction
  of 125
myalgic encephalomyelitis 23
myoma *see* fibroids
myths and facts about
  endometriosis 11–13

N-acetyl-L-cysteine (NAC) 165
NAPE *see* National Action Plan
  on Endometriosis (NAPE)
naproxen 66
National Aboriginal Community
  Controlled Health
  Organisation 240
National Action Plan on
  Endometriosis (NAPE) 29,
  44, 201, 259, 262, 263,
  268
National Endometriosis
  Clinical and Scientific
  Trials (NECST) Network
  259–260
National Health and Medical
  Research Council's
  (NHMRC) 93
National Women's Health
  Advisory Council 232, 274

natural therapies 287
NECST Network *see* National
  Endometriosis Clinical and
  Scientific Trials (NECST)
  Network
neuromodulators 67
neuromuscular reset 125
NHMRC *see* National Health and
  Medical Research Council's
  (NHMRC)
non-steroidal
  anti-inflammatories 66
Norton, Robyn 232
nuts and seeds 158

OCP *see* oral contraceptive
  pill (OCP)
OHNUT 147
O'Kane, Stephanie 110–114
omega-3 fatty acids 155,
  161, 162
omega-6 fatty acids 162
online peer support groups of
  endometriosis 282
oral contraceptive pill (OCP) 69,
  204
oral progestins 70
osteopathy for endometriosis
  123, 287
  cupping 124
  and dry needling 124
  holistic approach 124
  improved circulation and
    lymphatic drainage 123
  pain relief 123
  pelvic health 123
  stress reduction 123
ovarian cancer 289

risk of 25, 26
types of, associated with
  endometriosis 26
ovarian cysts 40, 83
ovarian endometriomas 4, 10
ovarian hyperstimulation 10, 95
ovarian reserve tests 93
over-the-counter medications 65
oxycodone 67
OxyContin 67
OxyNorm 67

pacing activities 128
pain, *see also* abdominal and
    pelvic pain, causes of
  chest 7
  defined 17
  during or after sex 6
  leg 6–7
  muscle pain relief, targeted 124
  pelvic 5
  pelvic *see* pelvic pain
  when toileting 6
painful intercourse 147
painful periods 5, 8, 9, 12, 30,
    35, 69, 142, 203–205, 207
pain relief 65, 72, 85, 123–125,
    192–193, 196, 204, 251
palmitoylethanolamide
    (PEA) 66
Panadeine Forte 66
Panadol 66
Panamax 66
Panamax Co 66
paracetamol 66
Parliamentary Friends of
    Endometriosis Awareness
    262–263

Paschimottanasana 177
patients' varied needs,
    supporting 110–114
PBS *see* Pharmaceutical Benefits
    Scheme (PBS)
PCOS *see* polycystic ovarian
    syndrome (PCOS)
PEA *see* palmitoylethanolamide
    (PEA)
pelvic examination 53–54, 251
pelvic health 123
pelvic inflammatory disease 22
pelvic pain 5, 17, 91, 164,
    173, 290
  causes of 20
    anaemia 23–24
    fatigue or low energy
      22–23
    fibroids (myoma or
      leiomyoma) 22
    inflammatory bowel
      disease 21
    interstitial cystitis 21
    mesenteric adenitis 21–22
    myalgic encephalomyelitis
      (chronic fatigue syndrome)
      23
    pelvic inflammatory
      disease 22
    polycystic ovarian syndrome
      (PCOS) 22
    small intestinal bacterial
      overgrowth (SIBO)
      20–21
    urinary tract infections 21
  clinics 263–264, 283
  endo's impact on the brain
    19–20

inflammation and nerves
    18–19
  persistent 204
Pelvic Pain Foundation of
    Australia 145, 147, 206
pelvic physiotherapy,
    115–117, 168
pelvic tilts 177
Period ImPact and Pain
    Assessment (PIPPA) 281
periods, menstrual 4, 85, 89, 90,
    103
  bleeding between 6
  cyclical *vs.* non-cyclical 4–5
  heavy 22
  irregular 5–6
  normal 5
  painful 5, 8, 9,
    12, 30, 35, 69, 142,
    203–205, 207
  progression 5
  severity 4
  timing and duration 4
Periods, Pain and Endometriosis
    Program (PPEP Talk) 206
peritoneal endometriosis 10
Pharmaceutical Benefits Scheme
    (PBS) 8
philanthropic donations, defined
    270
philanthropy, gift of 270
  Eden Foundation 271
  Lambert Initiative 271
  Wilson Foundation 270
physical activity and
    exercise 127
physical exam, preparing for
    52–53

physiotherapy 118–122, 290–291
pelvic 115–116, 168
phytoestrogens 163
pigeon pose (Eka Pada
Rajakapotasana) 178
Pilates 173
pill, prescription of 68
pill pack 71
PIPPA *see* Period ImPact and
Pain Assessment (PIPPA)
PMDD *see* premenstrual
dysphoric disorder
(PMDD)
polycystic ovarian syndrome
(PCOS) 22, 102
P party 208, 216
PPEP Talk *see* Periods, Pain and
Endometriosis Program
(PPEP Talk)
prebiotics 164
pregnancy and endometriosis
11, 12, 96, 103
premenstrual dysphoric disorder
(PMDD) 237
prescription medications 66
probiotics 164
progesterone-like hormones 70
progestin 68, 70
psychological support 127

QENDO 264, 275

RACGP *see* Royal Australian
College of General
Practitioners (RACGP)
Raising Awareness Tool for
Endometriosis (RATE)
32, 281

RANZCOG *see* Royal Australian
and New Zealand
College of Obstetricians
and Gynaecologists
(RANZCOG)
rASRM *see* Revised American
Society of Reproductive
Medicine (rASRM)
RATE *see* Raising Awareness Tool
for Endometriosis (RATE)
reclined bound angle pose
(Supta Baddha
Konasana) 177
relationships 139, 291
couples counselling 145–146
dads as endo supporters
141–142
daily life and responsibilities
147–148
educational resources 145
family planning 146
intimacy beyond sexuality 147
intimate 142–143
sex and intimacy 147
social isolation 148
support networks 148
relaxation exercises 128
reproductive leave 209–210
research funding, bias in 237–238
research on endometriosis
293–294
rest and recuperation (R&R) 187
cold water therapy 192
benefits of 192–193
cold shower at home 194
for endometriosis research at
the University of Adelaide
194–195

330 The Australian Guide to Living Well with Endometriosis

practice 193–194
safety precautions 195
fatigue and Spoon Theory 188–190
heat therapy 196
usage considerations 196
resveratrol 169
retrograde menstruation 13, 170
Revised American Society of Reproductive Medicine (rASRM) 8–9
Rombauts, Luk 95–97, 115, 269
Royal Australian and New Zealand College of Obstetricians and Gynaecologists (RANZCOG) 30, 54, 55, 67, 81
Royal Australian College of General Practitioners (RACGP) 40, 237
rye 158, 160
Ryeqo 70, 71, 91

Safe Work Australia 215
SCFAs *see* short-chain fatty acids (SCFAs)
school and work 201
About Bloody Time 211–212
adolescent girls 202–204
gendernomics 207
under-and unemployment, endo's impact on 209–210
UTERUSopia 208
UTERUSurper 208–209
Longitudinal Study of Teenagers with Endometriosis, Period

and Pelvic Pain (LongSTEPPP) 205
school education 206–207
teachers 204
workplace, endometriosis and 214
asking, art of 224
Australian workplace law 223–224
employee rights and workplace flexibility in Australia 216–217
employer obligations 226
research 214–215
workplace health and safety, responsibility for 215–216
school education 206–207
seated forward bend (Paschimottanasana) 177
selenium 169
self-care, lifestyle and 151–154
Setu Bandhasana 178
sex
and intimacy 147, 291
pain during or after 6
sex toys 147
sexually transmissible infections 22
shatavari 78
short-chain fatty acids (SCFAs) 165
shoulders 7
SIBO *see* small intestinal bacterial overgrowth (SIBO)
Simonis, Magdalena 58, 156
sleep hygiene 128
slippery elm 77

small intestinal bacterial overgrowth (SIBO) 20–21
social isolation 148
soy 162–163
Spoon Theory, fatigue and 188–190
stages/levels of endometriosis 8–10
stress management 128
stress reduction 123, 126, 193, 196
stretches, exercises and *see* exercises and stretches
stretching 128
superficial peritoneal endometriosis 10
superficial peritoneal lesions 4
supplements 169
support groups of endometriosis 281–282
support networks 148
Supta Baddha Konasana 177
surgery 81, 291–292
  hysterectomy 85
  laparoscopic 51, 81–85
swimming 173
symptoms of endometriosis 5, 31–32
  bleeding between menstrual periods 6
  digestive and gastrointestinal symptoms 7
  endo belly 7
  heavy menstrual bleeding or irregular periods 5–6
  leg pain 6–7
  pain during or after sex 6
  painful periods and cramps 5

pain when toileting 6
pelvic pain 5
symptoms GPs look for 40–41
sync set 147

Taylor, Jessica 264
teachers 204
team care arrangements 42
teenagers and young women+, endometriosis in 12
testing 30–31
tetrahydrocannabinol (THC) 72
TGA *see* Therapeutic Goods Administration (TGA)
THC *see* tetrahydrocannabinol (THC)
Therapeutic Goods Administration (TGA) 66, 274, 292
thermotherapy *see* heat therapy
thunder god vine 77
toileting, pain when 6
Tough, Caitlin 262
traditional and alternative options 76
  Chinese herbal medicine 77
  Indian Ayurvedic herbal therapies 77–78
  medicinal herbs 77
transvaginal ultrasound (TVUS) 55
treatment options 65
  analgesics 66
  hormone treatment options 67–69
  GnRH agonists 70
  GnRH antagonists 70–71

medicinal cannabis
71–72
oral contraceptive pill (OCP)
69
oral progestins 70
progesterone-like
hormones 70
neuromodulators 67
non-steroidal anti-
inflammatories 66
over-the-counter
medications 65
oxycodone 67
palmitoylethanolamide
(PEA) 66
prescription medications 66
traditional and alternative
options 76
Chinese herbal medicine 77
Indian Ayurvedic herbal
therapies 77–78
medicinal herbs 77
why are they prescribing the
pill? 68
turmeric 77
TVUS *see* transvaginal
ultrasound (TVUS)
Tylenol 66

ulcerative colitis 21
ultrasound 40, 54–55, 62
under-and unemployment,
endo's impact on 209–210
Uppal, Talat 35
urinary tract infections 21
UTERUSopia 208
UTERUSurper 208–209

vaginal hysterectomy 85
vaginal ring 92
vegetables 155, 157, 165
vitamin B12, 170
vitamin C 24, 169
vitamin D 155, 169
vitamin E 169

walking 173
walnuts 162
WCE *see* World Congress on
Endometriosis (WCE)
WEO *see* World Endometriosis
Organisations (WEO)
WES *see* World Endometriosis
Society (WES)
wheat 158–160, 164
whole grains 158
WHO *see* World Health
Organization (WHO)
Wilson Foundation
194, 270
Work Health and Safety Act 215
workplace 214
asking, art of 224
Australian workplace laws
223–224
employee rights and workplace
flexibility 216–217
employer obligations 226
endometriosis on women+
in 209
research 214–215
responsibility for workplace
health and safety,
215–216
rights and obligations in 292

Index **333**

workplace assistance program
210
World Congress on Endometriosis
(WCE) 95, 269
World Endometriosis
Organisations (WEO)
269–270, 280
World Endometriosis Society
(WES) 269

World Health Organization
(WHO) 268

Yazdani, Anusch 264
yoga 128, 173
yoghurt 165
young women+, endometriosis
in 12

zinc 169